How to Stay as Old as You Can

A New Script on Growing Healthier
Into Your 60s, 70s, 80s, and Even 90s

Doug Melody, Ph.D., CFT

outskirts
press

©HowToDieYoungAsOldAsYouCan

Doug Melody is a lifelong educator who has served in a variety of roles during a 46-year career in the profession, teaching at every level from kindergarten to graduate school and each grade level in between. With a Ph.D. in Educational Psychology, a dissertation completed in the area of sport performance, several certifications in the fitness field, a lifetime of working out in - literally - hundreds of gyms, and collaborating with scores of individuals in their quest to become more fully functioning human beings, Doug is now sharing his knowledge and experience with the hope that readers can begin to shape a new narrative on how to grow older in healthier ways. We can do better and this book is an attempt to explain both why and how we can do this.

Doug Melody, Ph.D, CPT
www.dougmelody.com

Table of Contents

PART 3 – IMPLEMENTING AN EFFECTIVE FUNCTIONAL FITNESS PLAN

PART 4 – ROLE MODELS & REFLECTIONS

Challenging the Script

We don't see things as they are.
We see them as we are.

LET ME ACKNOWLEDGE this up front: reading books about growing old is getting kind of old and yet here I am offering another one. So I wouldn't blame you for a moment if you're thinking this book is another gimmicky new-age plan that will add years to your life while juicing the quality of it, make you pain free, and even generate the kind of energy you want in order to throw your arms completely around life on your terms...all in just five easy minutes a day. It's not. It's definitely not new-age, and I'm not suggesting anything here that will be easy. You can be sure of this. No crystals or magnetic bracelets or magic potions will be offered in this book. What I am offering, though, is a time-tested plan that actually **will** add quality years to your life, reduce and even eliminate chronic pain, and produce a youthful energy with which to embrace life throughout a lifetime. But it will take more than five minutes a day to achieve this. Despite what many of us think, most all of us do have choices in our *"old age"*.

If you read this to its conclusion and I'm successful at constructing a persuasive argument in support of healthy aging, then I'm hoping you come to your senses and recognize the untapped potential inherent in each passing year that we're gifted in this life. I'm telling you that the script written for us regarding how we age is filled with misleading fallacies. *You can actually look forward to growing older.* Really. And why shouldn't you? You just need better directions, and I hope to provide them for you here on these pages.

Seriously - does the aging process really have to be a long, inexorable slog to inactivity, incompetence, incontinence, and even inattentiveness? Does being older mean enduring a life of chronic disease and disability? Is this all we have to look forward to as we age? I really don't believe so. I'm challenging the script currently in place that directs us on how we're expected to live out the third and fourth quarters of our lives, arguing that adherence to this false narrative is the root cause of our age-old beliefs about old age itself. There's a difference between actively **growing** older and passively getting older.

Having now personally completed 72 laps circling the sun, I'm writing to share with you that there is another lane available to most all of us. What we *"know"* to be aging is nothing more than a self-fulfilling prophecy grounded in misinformation and misconceptions. More accurately, our attitudes about the aging process make us brittle and broken long before our bones become so. The medical world, perhaps unknowingly, most certainly contributes to these misguided perceptions of aging, and so do many other established institutions in our culture, including our federal government. We belong to a culture that promotes these stereotypes, and I will explain how this is done in subsequent pages.

As already stated in the opening paragraph, it's just as important to emphasize that *"How To Die Young As Old As You Can"* is not an anti-aging treatise that promises to extend your lifespan (more on this later), nor is it a book that attempts to deliver on a pledge that you can lose 5 pounds in *"just 5 minutes a day"* of doing...whatever (there are enough bogus claims out there already that used to be the sole province of late night TV and have now been mainstreamed). Our healthcare system has indeed developed medicines and therapies that now extend the lifespan. It's our *health span* - the ability to engage with life in meaningful ways on our wished-for terms - that needs to expand in concert with these extra years the medical miracles are granting us. The average health span in the US is currently 66 years. But our lifespan is, on average, closer to 77. Do the math. We don't need to endure the last decade(s) of our lives in chronic pain and compromised health.

So, having cautioned you in the first paragraph that it won't be easy, these pages are meant to challenge as well as move you out of your comfort zone - physically, emotionally, cognitively, even spiritually - and to achieve this on a daily basis will require you **to become comfortable with being uncomfortable**. In the words of the poet E.E. Cummings, *"It takes courage to grow up and become who you really are."* It takes hard and smart work, no doubt. But it's well worth it with what the work gives back to us in return. We'll address this pain-pleasure relationship in a subsequent chapter.

Let me be up front here - aging is an unavoidable experience. There is no denying this and I'm not. But the multiple *effects* of aging are reversible and, if not completely avoidable, most definitely subject to a significant slowdown. There are several factors within our grasp that can assist in tapping the brakes to this inevitable decline—diet, sleep, regular visits to doctors, social networks—yet **the single most critical link to physical, emotional, and cognitive well-being is _physical activity_.** We require more *"moving experiences"* in our lives, some of which need to literally take our breath away. More about this will follow.

It takes courage, as Cummings reminds us, to age with grace and gratitude. A rare breed of older adults is already doing it, some of whom will be referred to in subsequent chapters here, proving that we can still generate the kind of energy necessary to live a full and active life right up to the *"final horn"*. George Burns, the lovable comedian, certainly did it, and he got it right when he said - *"You can't help getting older, but you don't have to get old."* Our goal should be **"to die young, as old as you can!"** He surely did.

And, finally for now, here's an invitation you may wish to consider from the distinguished Victorian poet, Robert Browning - *"Grow old along with me! The best is yet to be."* For most of us, it's a choice we make, knowingly or otherwise. How can you be so certain that you've already lived the best years of your life? The best may yet to be. Why not find out... before it's too late?

Really, what do you stand to lose by going for it?

PART ONE
PRESENTING MY CASE:
A BETTER SCRIPT

CHAPTER 1

An Uncommon Path

I am not a product of my circumstances.
I am a product of my decisions.

Stephen Covey

HERE'S SOME BACKGROUND on me to help you understand how and where I've travelled through life to arrive in this lane and space of what I believe is healthy aging.

It probably would be accurate to describe me as a contrarian. I have a rebellious streak that often has me exercise the belief that *"if it ain't broke, then we should damn well break it…and why wait?"*

Like you, I've had my pivotal moments. And, like you, it's how I've responded during these critical times that's made the difference in moving forward for me. After all, it's not just what happens to us that matters - it's how we *respond* to what happens that matters even more.

An acquired taste of mine along the way has been to remain comfortable with ambiguity while working at figuring out which turn to take next, especially when I'm injured. You can't choose prematurely simply to extinguish the stress of not knowing. Turns do matter. Right turns are better than wrong turns. Likewise, turns matter in that a life committed to growing requires them. So patience indeed must be my warrior strength. And yours, too.

I began my life in a gritty housing project in a lower middle-class suburb of Hartford, CT, experiencing the kind of childhood that would be so foreign to youngsters today. I played outdoors with other project kids while the sun was out and often crossed the nearby railroad tracks on our way to the public park that we viewed as our own backyard. No adults were necessary to organize and supervise these games…we could simply be kids, resolving conflicts and figuring it all out on our own.

I lived with both my parents, my older brother by five years and younger sister by three. It's worth noting here that most of the project kids were my brother's age and so I was always needing to *"play up"* whenever pick-up games were arranged…which was typically all day and every day. Having to compete with and against the big kids in all likelihood laid the groundwork for me feeling the need to prove myself time and again as I moved through high school and college. In a way, I've adopted the mindset of *"playing up"* to this day, except that I'm now focused on playing as if I'm younger than the fallacious narrative tells me I should be.

My decisions for attending both high school and college were reduced to one factor - basketball. The game grew on me as I tagged along with my dad to high school and college games that he refereed in my childhood days and it eventually became my passion in my younger life, one that simultaneously gave me a chance to lose myself in the moment of the game while dreaming of a future with bright lights and playing on the big stage. This eventually led me to a local Catholic high school that specialized in winning state championships. We delivered on that specialty by capturing one in 1968 - my senior year.

Upon graduating, I moved up the road to the The University of Connecticut (UConn), chasing a childhood dream to play for the program there, a team that I had followed religiously as a young kid growing up in the Nutmeg State and whose players I idolized while hoping to be like them there one day. This was the big stage I referred to moments ago. It turned out to be a decision that would impact me for the rest of my life and one that, in a very surreal way, provided the final impetus to write this book (more on this in a moment).

I showed up at UConn in the fall of 1968 pumped about playing for State U right in front of me when I was blindsided by members of the Students for a Democratic Society in the student union while picking up first-year student materials along with my freshman beanie. I was handed a leaflet that was disturbingly disorienting…during my student orientation. The message was a <u>W</u>(hat)<u>T</u>(he)<u>F</u>(uck) moment for me - don't trust the government, the church, or anything else I've been led to believe is true.

Wait, what? This is my welcome to college? Can I at least wear my beanie?

In hindsight, it was a prelude to the chaos and confusion that erupted on our campus and just about every other across the country in the few years that followed during the late sixties and early seventies. Recall Vietnam, Kent State, the assassinations of Martin Luther King and Robert Kennedy, the drug culture, race conflicts. This wasn't your typical party time on campus or spring break at Daytona Beach. And I don't remember any part of this being in my childhood dream. So, go figure, my dream soon became a nightmare amidst bomb scares in gymnasiums and sit-ins of administration buildings, with the wonderful world I thought I knew becoming incredulously dark and confusing. It brought to light for me a phrase on a poster I recall that hung in the art room at my high school - *"If sometimes you don't get lost, there's a chance you may never find your way"*. I was clearly lost, and desperately needing to find my way.

If the liberal arts are meant to encourage *"free thinking"*, then I most certainly experienced a liberal arts education while in college. Much of what I was raised to believe - trust our government leaders, worship faithfully at the foot of the church alter, all people are created equal - was suddenly called into question, and the *"truth"* I thought I had known seemed like a pile of horse shit now. The counter-culture was taking shape, the drug scene was ramping up, and writers like Carlos Castaneda were offering alternative perspectives for me. It was during this time when I developed what I feel was, and still remains for me, a healthy skepticism about *"accepted truths"* that I've carried with me since those formative years.

Eventually, I found my way...and it's happened to be a way other than the *"normal"* path. It's been the proverbial road less traveled: a perfectly uncommon path for a contrarian like me.

So my dream-turned-nightmare experience at UConn at least instilled in me a questioning spirit that has pissed off a fair number of people along the way (challenging the status quo can do that, right?) but, nevertheless, has served me well through my adulthood - and I dare say others around me, too. I share this with you because, as it relates to this writing, my healthy skepticism has had me question the beliefs and expectations we have of what aging is supposed to be and has led me to **my** truth about how we can live healthier years into our sixties, seventies, eighties and beyond.

Moving forward, I devoted forty-six years to the profession of education, serving in a variety of roles as a classroom teacher, coach, counselor, advisor, department supervisor, regional director, undergraduate and graduate instructor, and personal fitness coach.

Work stress seemed to mount as my work responsibilities increased, and I'm sure the challenges/frustrations I grappled with along the way were common, garden-variety issues that most people deal with on a regular basis. Here's an important point, though - *it's **how** we choose to deal with these issues that matters going forward far more than the issues themselves.* How I chose to manage this increasing stress that was compounded by an expanding family (read: more kids) and caring for a parent who eventually moved in with us (the sandwich generation moment) has unquestionably been a critical factor in my self-care. As Stephen Covey reminds us, we're products of our decisions and not our circumstances... more on this later.

I broke a lot in over four decades during my professional career. Hopefully, I built back better. For the record, I'm not done breaking. I sincerely hope this book breaks apart the falsehoods about aging and we build back a much healthier way to grow older moving forward.

For me, my daily workouts have been (and continue to be) my prescription pills for stress and anxiety. Let's be real here - it has never been easy to do, especially during a stretch of time (with young kids) that had me getting up with the birds in the dark. But it has always been worth doing because it re-centers me while getting rid of the toxins picked up during the course of the previous day. The more often I commit to exercise, the easier it is to do. This is how habits are formed, as you will see in Chapters 12 and 13. At 72, it's still an integral part of my day. I mostly do in my seventies what I was doing in my fifties because I've continued doing it all these years and modified where appropriate when it would have been so much easier to remain fixed to the recliner, remind myself that I'm getting old and *"can't be doing this shit anymore at my age"*, crack open a beer, and pop a Xanax. Besides, the beer tastes so much better AFTER the workout if I decide to enjoy one. Xanax?...no thanks.

As for injuries, illnesses, and setbacks, I've had my collection but realize I've also been fortunate in avoiding those that can end life prematurely or alter it dramatically. Aside from normal sprains, muscle tears, broken bones, back spasms, a herniated disk, bronchitis, pneumonia, hernia surgery, drop foot (for seven months) from a pinched perineal nerve, arthritis, bouts of transitory depression, shingles and - of course - Covid, there have been a few setbacks that have knocked me on my ass and from which, not surprisingly, I've gained the most insight and eventual strength. I will refer to some of these at various points in the book.

One I'm sharing now served as the tipping point for me to write this and has brought me full-circle back to my childhood. I injured my whole left side catching a large man (240 pounds) from falling who I was spotting during a personal training session. It happened in the first week of 2022. My fascia, back, shoulder, obliques, quadriceps, psoas…everything on my left side was inflamed and incredibly painful. Here's where it comes full circle - the person I happened to be spotting was a former UConn basketball player I watched when I was a young child. It just made me wonder how one who was such an accomplished athlete in adolescence and early adulthood could morph into a shadow of his former self? How does this happen? This mishap ignited the desire for me to share my experience with how I've grown older and to provide research data that backs it up. The injury, by the way, took a full nine weeks for me to recover from completely…and with a ton of work, some of which included massage and physical therapy as well as acupuncture. Most of it was exercising patience and trusting in my own recovery plan (this is what I mean by being comfortable in ambiguity). I wish to note that my recovery did not include prescription or over-the-counter painkillers (there will be more about the adverse effects of painkillers in a subsequent chapter). I trusted the process and the professionals assisting me. It was a decision I made in the face of these circumstances. I'm so thankful for my full recovery.

For the record, I'm stronger now (yes - at 72) in my upper body than I was in my teens and early twenties because I only began strength training in my late twenties. Any athlete my age will recall the forbidden nature of weight-lifting back in the sixties - whatever the sport. In hindsight, this made about as much sense as advising pregnant women in the 1950s to smoke cigarettes in order to control their weight. As for my lower body, the strength is there, but I have no illusions of grabbing the basketball rim again anytime soon.

A few other important areas of emphasis for me - I haven't eaten red meat since 1977, haven't consumed soda and have significantly reduced foods that contain refined sugar and other sweeteners in a similar length of time, have refrained from fried foods (with some exceptions) for at least four decades, and I began occasionally using CBD legally in 2018 as a sleep and recovery aid (I will address the endocannaboid system in a later chapter). As for supplements, my daily regimen includes 3000 mg of glucosamine, 2200 mg of chondroitin, 400 mg of saw palmetto, 400 mg of pygeum, a tablespoon of collagen, 400 mg of CoQ10, and 100 mg of Boswellia. In addition, my one prescription added last year is 10mg of a statin. All, in their own unique ways, have aided in my healthy aging.

I am simply sharing this for those of you who may be interested. It should not be viewed as a prescription nor a recommendation. You can decide for yourself to what degree any of this makes sense for you in the context of your life. Know that it's not all-or-nothing here. Various degrees of moderation may work for you. Each of us needs to choose what we're willing to *"sacrifice"* on our way to optimal health and well-being...to being the **best** version of ourselves that we can possibly be.

I believe it's still possible to be a red-blooded American without having to chow down red-blooded meat, fried foods, sugar-laced soda, or heavily-processed fast food *on a daily basis* - as strange and eccentric as this may sound to you. In fact, given the rising costs of healthcare in our country, one might argue it's a patriotic duty to protect our own health and well-being in order to keep government-funded healthcare coverage in check...because we all know that, if left underchecked, expanding waistlines along with the clogged arteries and illnesses associated with this expansion will eventually balloon into unsustainable fixed costs that will surely overburden the federal budget.

Maybe we should be invoking the words of John F. Kennedy, who challenged the American people back in the early 1960s with this remark - *"Don't ask what your country can do for you, ask what you can do for your country."* We can start by taking better care of ourselves. This book is designed to help you do this while becoming the best version of yourself...today and going forward.

CHAPTER 2

Is Age Really Just A Number?

"What You Think, You Become"

Unknown

I HAVE THIS phrase posted on a wall in my home gym that reads *"What You Think, You Become"* and it reminds me to check in on my thought pattern each time I enter the space. Think about it - the messages we play back in our heads help to tell us who we are. At 72, what am I *supposed to think* as a septuagenarian, according to the *"scripture"*? I could care less because I pay no attention to it. Most of the time. And you shouldn't either. Most of the time. But do you? John Milton, a name you may recall from your high school British Literature course, said it this way - *"The mind is its own place and in itself can make a heaven of hell or a hell of heaven."* Many of us can probably admit that we sometimes do this to ourselves in counterproductive ways. But if we can make ourselves miserable with what we're thinking, shouldn't we be able to do the opposite as well? Can we create our own heavenly spaces? Legally?

Let's take a closer look at this personally constructed reality we create for ourselves, consciously or otherwise. However old you currently are, take a moment to consider this - **today** you're as old as you've ever been and, guess what, you will never be any younger going forward than you are - **today**.

Obviously, you know where you've been (although that's open to interpretation and change - just call yourself a re-visionist historian). Now imagine what your future self may look like in say…5, 10, 25 years? What are you thinking when you imagine this preview of coming attractions? What're you seeing? Do you exert *any* control over how this will play out? Seriously, think about how *your* perceptions influence the person you eventually become later on. Will you let a number dictate who that is, as author Richard J. Leider warns us we may do?

> *"The trouble is, when a number—your age— becomes your identity, you've given away your power to choose your future."*

You already know that any reference in today's media to the aging will likely provide a depressing image (unless you count the 50-something-year-old female celebrity posing on social media with her rock-hard abs) and a glance at the typical older individual probably doesn't have you wishing for those *"golden years"* any time soon. God help anyone 65 or older during the pandemic, the age we repeatedly heard that suddenly spiked our chances of dying or otherwise suffering horribly from that worldwide bug we've been dealing with these past few years. What is it about this number that marks danger for the virus and is a digit that has been used elsewhere as well for a reference point - i.e., the first federally-established full retirement age (it's now 66 and climbing)?

Actually, the Committee on Economic Security that was established way back in 1935 recognized both the harsh economic reality of forced retirement and the absolute social necessity to keep the young employed. So the Committee eventually settled on 65 as the marker of *"retirement"* age for its economic feasibility. At the time, life expectancy at birth - get ready for this - was 58. Of course, there are other numbers along the chronological continuum that have been assigned arbitrary significance, too. And then we have our own personal ones.

For better or worse, we routinely use chronological age to mark various passages through life; from which age group we're able to compete in with sports, or when we're responsible enough to first drive, legally buy booze, or vote in an election, to when we can collect social security or begin to score on those farcical senior citizen deals. And then there are the regularly suggested medical exams and booster shots we should get at yada-yada numerical age along the lifespan. Still another glaring example surfacing these days is the recent call for age limits on certain positions in government - like, say President or Supreme Court Justice or U.S. Senator. No small-potato targets here. (Some think the current President is cause for concern. And others believe a certain Senator from California is too. Still, I wonder what Warren Buffet is thinking...or Mick Jagger, for that matter.)

So this metric - chronological age - gets baked into our consciousness early and continues on slow cook throughout our lives. It's certainly convenient to use digits as this eliminates any subjectivity otherwise involved. The number is the number...except it isn't - and we all know it. It's the implied and ascribed significance of the digits that often matters far more. We allow a number to become our identity....to define who we are. And this definition of ourselves directs our behavior.

If you're looking for proof on how much of how we feel is fueled by *how we're expected to feel,* then a recent study published in *JAMA Network Open* may provide it. A research group from both the University of Oklahoma and the University of Michigan examined the data from a survey of more than 2,000 people between the ages of 50 and 80 that was drawn from the *National Poll On Healthy Aging* and uncovered a strong relationship between a person's internalized (meaning...they believed it) exposure to ageism and their overall health. The higher a subject's score on a measure of everyday ageism experiences, the more likely they are to be in poor physical or mental health, to have more chronic health issues and to exhibit symptoms of depression. But which comes first - poor health or negative perceptions of aging?

A basics Statistics course teaches us that correlation doesn't necessarily mean causation - you know, like just because your favorite team wins each time you watch it play while in your favorite chair wearing your favorite uniform jersey and they happen not to win when you don't, well it must mean...right? Kind of. But not really.

Still, although the study can't show cause and effect (do one's perceptions cause the behavior or vice versa?), the authors of this study note that the relationship between ageism and health/well-being needs to be examined more closely, with a shift in focus to creating programs that encourage positive expectations of health and well-being among older adults. *"These findings raise the question of whether aging-related health problems reflect the adverse influences of ageism and present the possibility that anti-ageism efforts could be a strategy for promoting older adult health and well-being,"* cautions first author Julie Ober Allen, Ph.D., MPH, Department of Health and Exercise Science, University of Oklahoma, Norman. This book you're currently reading is designed to do just that.

What might happen if we began to view our future selves more favorably and to envision our future lives with optimism? Would it make a difference if we began to shift the narrative on aging to a more positive outlook? Would older folks experience aging differently?

A fresh analysis dives even deeper into these issues and uses the *Everyday Ageism Scale* constructed by the aforementioned research team to further explore this correlation. The scale spits out a score based on a subject's answers to ten questions about their own personal experiences and perceptions with growing older. In the study of everyday aging, *ninety-three percent* of the older adults surveyed reported that they often experienced at least one of the ten forms of ageism addressed in the survey. The most prevalent form reported by *almost eighty percent* was agreeing with the statement that **"having health problems is part of getting older"**.

So here you go. What we think, we become. Would it instead be more accurate to say that having health problems is part of the human condition across the life span and not just for the aged? Granted, we may become more susceptible to infirmities with every successive lap around the sun. But health problems are the result of infections and metabolic conditions more than aging. Health problems are more often caused by unhealthy lifestyles rather than some random number.

Still more, *sixty-five percent* of the older adults reported that they consistently notice, hear or read satirical jokes about older people as well as messages that older adults are unattractive or undesirable. I'm sure you've heard your share of these already, and maybe even made a contribution or two to the growing list of jokes. This kind of *"internalized"* ageism also included agreeing with the statements that feeling lonely, or feeling depressed, sad or worried, are part of getting older. It's worth mentioning here that the study doesn't indicate duration of time with regard to those feelings. Each is a feeling that's natural when experienced in short durations - a few days to a couple of weeks - and becomes problematic when felt for any longer.

It seems like how much money we're raking in annually, what academic degrees we've collected, and where we plant our roots can also affect our perceptions of aging. Respondents who reported lower levels of income or education as well as those who lived in rural areas had average ageism scores that were much higher as compared to others. Older adults who said they spend four hours or more each day in front of the television, surfing the web or reading magazines had higher scores than those with less exposure to such media. This is likely the case because of the stereotypes commonly appearing on television, on line, and in print media. And, it's a whole lot of sitting on your ass...which is now compared closely to smoking cigarettes with regard to the adverse effects on our health.

When the researchers examined each subject's score and compared these scores to what the same subjects had reported about their own health - including self-rated physical and mental health and the number of chronic conditions - those who had higher *Everyday Ageism* scores were more likely to have disclosed that their general physical and/or mental health were fair or poor, reported having more chronic health conditions as well as more signs of depression...*which they attribute to aging*...and which may more accurately be attributed to expectations. You'll soon see why.

Many of us surely remember how we longed for reaching the sweet age of 16 or 18 or 21. But are we longing in the same way about reaching 50? How about 65? 80? What about those numbers that end in "0"? How old is old, anyway? And how powerful are those expectations we hold for our future years? Already we've seen in this one study shared here how our perceptions can shape our actions. We've seen that what we think, we become. View the aging experience as one in which you expect serious health issues waiting for you as you grow older and sure enough you increase the likelihood of your predictions being spot on.

I'm writing to say there is another way to think about how we age and, concomitantly, another way to experience our later years other than the current narrative we're given to follow. As I stated at the start of this chapter, I don't pay any attention to the traditional narrative most of the time and you shouldn't, either. The research results presented here reveal the impact our thinking has on our reality.

We'll explore possible answers to the aforementioned questions and others as we move forward. While we're doing this, though, we need to regularly remind ourselves that the danger for us lies not in what we don't know, but in what we think we know that just isn't the case. What's this mean? It means we may need to admit we're wrong. So we should prepare ourselves for resistance to any conflicting views, ideas, and the like (we tend to protect our *"truth"*). Initially, we resist alternative views because they cause cognitive dissonance (confusion/brain fog) and we don't like how that feels. What normal human being would?

Here's my tough-love counselor advice - **deal with it**. Be a grown-up and stay in that space of ambiguity for as long as it takes to find your next course of action. Change is uncomfortable, but often necessary. We all know it's not easy to change course, nor is starting over any easier. So, for too many of us, it's instead much more convenient to remain comfortably stuck in our known misery rather than confront the discomforting fear of the unknown.

To move requires a leap of faith. To grow, we have to trust… growth only occurs outside one's comfort zone. And what this means is that we'll need to prepare ourselves to be uncomfortable because this is what we feel when we move outside those cozy boundaries. I'll remind you again and again throughout this book that you'll need to get comfortable with being uncomfortable. What you're doing is expanding those limits, increasing that space.

If we're going to re-write the script on growing older, it's critical for us to first look more closely at what it means to age and how we are currently experiencing it.

CHAPTER 3

Why Do We Age?

I cannot see/ I cannot pee/ I cannot chew/ I cannot screw/ My memory shrinks/ My hearing stinks/ No sense of smell/ I look like hell/ My body's drooping/ Have trouble pooping/ The Golden Years have come at last/ The Golden Years can kiss my ass.

Dr. Seuss - The Golden Age poem

DR. SEUSS PRETTY much sums it up for us, doesn't he? Live long enough and all of the the above awaits us. It's hardly anything to die for.

But why is this? Why do we age? Why do we even *have* to age? Why can't we just live forever? These questions are as old as time and have been contemplated for centuries, but the formal study of aging is a relatively new science and it's only been in the last fifty years that researchers have become really serious about doing a deep dive into it.

Most of the research concentrates on ways to extend life, to add years if not decades to our lifespans. A quick Google search on the concept of aging will deliver a whole host of links that offer anti-aging advice, from magical elixirs to magnetic bracelets. Each link, in its own way, seems to be offering a *"cure"* for growing older. But wait a second - if it's a cure we're seeking, then what does this say about aging in and of itself?

If you're thinking what I'm thinking, cures are typically for illness and disease. So is this how we're supposed to view the aging process - as a dreaded sickness? Well, don't we kind of already?

We may, as we already observed with the research presented in the previous chapter, but we shouldn't - according to author Ashton Appleton, who believes that *"aging is not a disease, otherwise living would be a disease, but you can't make money off satisfaction."* She makes no distinction between living and aging - they are one and the same. After all, if you're living, then you're aging. So, if you subscribe to Appleton's thought process, we need to manufacture disease and illness in order to make money off the magical elixirs and magnetic bracelets we've developed to *"cure"* them. What a business model. And what unwitting participants we can be in support of this paradigm.

The mystery of aging has even garnered its share of attention in recent years from a few obscenely wealthy human beings who are exploring ways in which we can become… immortal. This book isn't focused upon adding years to our lives: **it's about adding quality.** What good is another decade added if we're experiencing it in chronic pain and limited movement? No thank you. Add a decade while preserving

functional fitness? Sign me up. Now. It's the gist of this book...
increasing our **health** span and not our lifespan.

So let's get serious and describe aging more formally than
Dr. Seuss has done for us. Aging refers to the *inevitable* physi-
ological changes that occur in a lifetime; our skin shrivels, our
skeletons shrink, our bones get brittle, muscles weaken, our
brains become foggy - you don't need more reminders. Dr. Seuss
is actually on point so far. Ask a physician why we age and each
is likely to provide an answer based upon their area of expertise
(not unlike why you may be suffering from just about any ailment). Given this, you can imagine the multitude of theories that
exist to help us understand why decay awaits us all.

That said, it shouldn't be any surprise then that there have
been several attempts to make sense of this phenomenon of
aging and there are currently about 300 theories that try to
explain it, with no uniform agreement by scientists on any
particular one, according to a Russian biogerontologist by the
name of Zhores Medvedev. But Steven Austad, another biogerontologist at the University of Alabama at Birmingham, believes that one explanation appears to have taken hold across
virtually all the theories as the most plausible argument for
why we age:

> *"Reproduction is the name of the game. Basically, we
> age because it's not in nature's best interest to per-
> fectly repair our bodies. The main thing is to keep us
> reproductive as long as possible, and then let our bod-
> ies deteriorate."*

So, in essence, we exist to procreate. When we're no longer pros at creating, then there's no need to keep us around. We become excess baggage to the human race. Don't let the door hit you in the...

Without getting too technical and lost in the details here, the few hundred explanations that currently exist tend to be grouped into any of three categories: **"wear and tear" theories, genetic mutation theories,** or **programmed aging theories.** The first believe that aging is the result of a slow meltdown of the body over time that's caused by both internal and external triggers. The second group resembles the first with regard to our cells eventually malfunctioning from exposure to toxins while the third, programmed aging theories, maintain that aging is a process that's wired into the body by evolutionary means to intentionally close down repair mechanisms and, thus, allow the body to age and eventually die. Ain't nothing we can do about it, according to the programmed aging group of theorists. It's also quite possible that an explanation of why we age may borrow tenets from each of the grouped theories. In other words, we'll all eventually - if we're lucky and don't perish prematurely - experience the wear and tear of our cellular structures as a consequence of living and breathing and our lifestyle choices, no matter what we do or don't do. It's just that the first two groups seem to suggest a personal degree of control in the pace we take to our eventual obsolescence. The third doesn't.

Regarding this preset programming (programmed aging theories), the thinking here is that each of us will eventually take an involuntary turn giving it up for the greater good. In other words, the preservation of the community (in Darwinian terms) takes precedence over the individual. This is why the individual weakens and eventually perishes. We're just being good team players. Longevity influencer Josh Mitteldorf explains it this way in **Cracking the Aging Code.**

"Though aging is bad for the individual, it is important for the community. Aging creates opportunities for the young and thus it promotes population turnover for adaptive change. Another communal benefit of aging is the stabilization of populations. Aging levels the death rate so individuals don't all die at once, as in famines and epidemics."

(So here's your argument for implementing the age restrictions on the Presidency, etc. mentioned in the previous chapter. It also supports the rationale provided by the Council on Economic Security back in 1935).

Generally speaking, according to the experts, that pretty much explains the programmed theories - it's all in the proverbial cards for each of us and we kind of have to just wait our turn to fold. So let's take a closer peek at a few of the other theories of aging that may shed light on what we can do to decelerate this process.

This group of *"wear and tear"* and genetic mutation theories on why we age may sound familiar to us in that references have frequently been made to these theories by the media in recent years. Internal and external elements like environmental pollution, toxins, cosmic radiation, as well as insidious bacteria and viruses wreak havoc and create errors at the basic cellular level. *A good portion of these pollutants are the result of choices we make* and the rest we can chalk up to the basic costs of living (one of the costs, believe it or not, is breathing). These errors, in turn, muck up the body's natural repair system and can eventually lead to serious illnesses and infirmities...like cancer, Alzheimer's, infections, and heart disease. These are all too familiar to us.

You've probably heard of free radicals. They were the rage several years back when marketers realized there was a treasure trove to be made on anti-oxidants. So the *Free Radical Theory of Aging* emerged as a member of the *"wear and tear"* paradigm. This is likely the oldest theory in the group, having originated in the 1950s and it peaked in popularity around 15 years ago. It's since fallen out of favor among many scientists for at least a few reasons - there are several antioxidants like beta carotene, vitamin A, and vitamin E that provide zero protection from free radicals and actually may promote death; anti-oxidants do nothing for heart disease; and some studies suggest that an increase in free radicals actually extends life. So the free radical theory of aging was kicked to the curb early this century and others have surfaced in the wake of its demise. All this said, you should still eat your blueberries and other anti-oxidants because they're good for you in other ways...and they taste delicious. They just may not be knocking off free radicals like the Pac Man we thought they were.

Another to surface was the *DNA Damage Theory of Aging* and this one seems to be logical in that we know DNA and genetics have a lot to do with who we are. So it would make intuitive sense that our own personal DNA influences how we age. But how influential is it really? The DNA damage theory, originally sprouting in the 1960s, hypothesizes that as we age, the cellular repair mechanisms that usually fix DNA strands break, cross-linkages get screwed up, and transcription errors stop working as well as they once did. This results in DNA damage—which is caused by everything from random copying errors to radiation to those free radicals we discussed above—and the junk slowly starts to build up in our cells. It simply seems to be the cost of living we incur for breathing, as noted moments ago, in such a *"radical"* environment.

As this DNA damage accumulates and worsens in millions of different cells in our bodies, several of them either die, cease to function properly, or morph into zombie senescent cells that turn into awful neighbors by emitting destructive signals to their nearby healthy cells. The net effect of all this is that as we age our bodies becomes less functional, weaker, and more susceptible to disease. I'm still hearing you, Dr. Seuss. It sounds all too familiar...according to the traditional script.

The *DNA Damage Theory of Aging* also has a decent amount of research to support it, including outcomes that demonstrate centenarians have elevated levels of DNA repair enzymes in their bodies and that mice with mutations that prevent them from sufficiently repairing DNA damage actually tending to age more rapidly. Moreover, certain diseases in humans related to premature aging, like progeria, are triggered by DNA damage and result in people who are chronologically young experiencing many of the symptoms of old age, including wrinkles, cardiovascular disease, and bone strength issues.

One more theory worth considering from this set of *"wear and tear theories"* is the *Epigenetic Theory,* also known as the

Information Theory of Aging. This is a fairly new perspective that has been proposed and promoted by such prominent life-extension researchers as Harvard's David Sinclair and Steve Horvath of UCLA, the creator of the epigenetic clock for measuring biological age (more on bio-markers and the clock in another chapter). Similar to the DNA damage theory of aging, scientists still distinguish enough differences to consider this a distinct and separate position. Including the epigenome is a major difference in large part because of the impact our chosen lifestyles can have on it.

According to the *Epigenetic Theory of Aging,* damage to your epigenome—how your DNA is packaged and expressed—causes us to weaken, become more frail and more susceptible to the infirmities all too often related to aging. The epigenome plays a critical role by dictating the identity of each cell and by expressing or suppressing specific genes. It's sometimes referred to as a switchboard operator (I remember those operators. Do you?) who turns switches off and on. A skin cell, for example, will express certain genes but not others, while a heart cell will express and suppress an entirely different set of genes.

Here's where it can get ugly. As we've already learned from similar theories, damage to our cells is caused by toxins and radiation and this adversely impacts the epigenome. When this happens, cells start to lose their *"identities"* and *"forget"* what kind of cells they're supposed to be. It's like that switchboard operator getting confused and starting to mix up the connections. If this identity confusion isn't corrected soon enough - meaning that the damaged cells aren't repaired - then heart cells may start to act like skin cells and vice versa, igniting all sorts of problematic issues that can eventually lead to cell death or senescence. When cells start misbehaving, trouble can be just up the road.

Having said all this, the *epigenetic theory* provides pretty encouraging promise in helping to understand the phenomenon of aging. Unlike our DNA, which is locked in at the moment of conception and doesn't really change throughout our lives, our epigenome on the other hand is constantly changing and is actually relatively easy to modify and here's why: it*'s our lifestyle habits, from smoking to drinking to exercise to diet that have been shown to influence and alter our epigenetics* - **factors well within our control to manage.**

Rachel Burger, a writer and co-founder of *Longevity Advice,* describes it in this way - *"Your DNA can't change—think of it like the script of King Lear. No matter in which playhouse you might watch the drama, the lines all remain uniform. However, the director, the actors, the stagehands—your epigenetics, to continue the metaphor—might change. If you eat poorly and exercise irregularly, your DNA's performance might seem more akin to a high school production than a masterpiece produced by London's Royal Shakespeare Company."*

In effect, then, Burger is arguing that we serve as our own directors and actors, delivering on the lines of DNA given to us in this experience we call life. We stage our own productions. We produce and direct our own lives. We're mostly in control. Do you want this responsibility?

If it's realistic hope we're searching for (and why wouldn't we?), then this most recent theoretical position offers the kind of promise in understanding why we age as we do and that we exercise an *imperfect* control over the pace of our aging (actually by exercising, as you'll soon see). There appears to be a direct cause-and-effect relationship between lifestyle choices and gene expressions. Moreover, this relationship now makes the common go-to explanation known as *"I can't help it, it's in my genes"* a weak excuse. The thinking that if you *"know a person's genes, you know the person"* disappears. We actually may be able to help it. Genes do control. But it turns out that they can also *be* controlled...in both healthy and unhealthy ways. We actually are able to wield much more control than we thought otherwise, albeit an imperfect control that it is. How much? If the general consensus among experts is that nature and nurture carry relatively equal weight in determining who we become, then the control we exert over our gene expression accounts for as much as fifty percent of the pace we keep towards our eventual decay. The ball, it appears, is in our proverbial court. The script is in our hands.

Considering the possibilities of control we exert in our pace to old age as we know it then, it may actually be more accurate for Dr. Seuss to shout *"kiss my ass"* to aging prematurely and the traditional script that encourages it. It appears that, if we want to, we actually can exert more control over the play that unfolds for us going forward. Let's next develop the notion of **how** we age to piggyback what we've learned thus far.

CHAPTER 4

How Do We Age?

**"When it comes to staying young,
a mind-lift beats a face-lift any day."**

Marty Buccella

SO WE SHOULD have a sense by now of why we age and that we actually may be able to wield more control over it than we previously thought with the pace of our eventual demise. Knowing this, we should naturally be able to exercise at least some control over *how* we age. Let's see if this is the story.

Each of us has our own experience with this aging thing and, as we've likely observed, it can be quite different for even individuals of the same chronological age. When asked about our age, we often respond with *"Well, I feel like"*... That's what it is - a feeling. Sometimes *I feel* like my chrono-logical age (which is still a subjective interpretation) - mostly in the first hour of the day when I resemble a tractor trailer exiting from a rest stop. As the sun brightens and the day un-folds, *I feel* younger and younger, especially after my workout.

I eventually work my way up to the speed I want. But what I'm sharing here is anecdotal information.

It's important, before going any further with this topic of how we age, to differentiate aging as we seem to know it from healthy aging, with the latter being the primary focus of this book. The World Health Organization defines healthy aging *as the process of developing and maintaining the functional ability that enables well-being in older age.* Strongly implied in this definition is the emphasis upon functional fitness and extension of one's *health* span. With this in mind, there have been efforts to formally study how we age, and one in particular has attracted a significant amount of attention.

The Baltimore Longitudinal Study of Aging (BLSA) is recognized as one of the world's longest continuing studies on aging and is America's oldest of its kind. Launched in 1958 when gerontology was in its infancy, the study continues today as researchers still enroll participants who are 20 or older and monitor them for the duration of their lives.

The original purpose of the study was to discover markers of aging, with the hope that specific biological markers could be identified at established points along the chronological continuum of a lifespan. Those who participate agree to complete an extensive battery of health tests and measures every three years throughout their lives, with these tests including blood work, physical tests for mobility, cognitive testing, and body composition. To date, there have been over 3200 participants. The BLSA has produced one of the largest and most comprehensive data sets available and, after 60+ years of study, researchers have concluded that aging is a whole lot different than we've been led to believe.

Aging, according to the BLSA findings, is highly variable and *we all age differently*. Moreover, *the older we get the more variation there is*. If this isn't enough to confound you, researchers have found there isn't one single marker for aging, but that *there are several strong predictors of how individuals do age*.

As one might imagine, the researchers may have been surprised with these findings. The one conclusive result was that the outcomes were *in*conclusive relative to what they were may have been looking to discover. There was absolutely no consistency in the data as it related to the passage of time. Let's repeat the findings - *the ways in which individuals age are as varied as there are people in the study*. There is simply no uniform way to age. Period.

So how do we age then? It seems like this experience of growing older can get very personal. It also means that we don't march to the same drum beat as we parade through life; some age as a factor greater than one (you may be one chronological year older but also may have aged *biologically* by *more* than one year), some the same as, and still others as a factor less than one. This translates into some people looking older than their age should *"reveal"* while others seem to look much younger. Then there are those who are simply *"acting their age"*, resembling precisely what they're supposed to look like.

While this study is ongoing and there remains much more to learn, three significant conclusions can be extrapolated from the BLSA research outcomes thus far. **One** is this - changes that occur with normal aging don't inevitably cause such diseases as diabetes, hypertension, or dementia. *The several disorders that typically show up in old age are a result of disease processes and not normal aging.* **Two** - there is no such thing as a single absolute chronological timetable of human aging. It doesn't exist. *We all age differently.* **And how about this research finding** - with regard to change and development, *there are more differences among older people than there are among younger people.*

Put a group of sixty-five 65 year-olds in a room and you'll get 65 different variations on what it means to be 65 years old (which raises my ire when reflecting upon that number - 65 - and the attention it received during the lockdown). And these differences will be greater than the comparisons found among the group of 21-year-olds you assembled in the room right next door. A combination of lifestyle, genetics, and disease processes impact the rate of aging between and within all individuals. Take note of the first factor mentioned - **lifestyle**.

So the BLSA informs us that how we age is highly personal. The research findings from this study also point to the two strongest predictors that correlate with healthy aging - *our personally-held attitudes toward getting/growing older and our ability to physically move during middle age.* What's this mean? Quite simply, it means that the more positive we are about aging while in our 40s and 50s the better we are likely to age. There are those who think that growing older sucks and those who don't. You're much better off belonging to the second group (remember - *What You Think, You Become*). Haven't we already seen this in the study using the *Everyday Ageism Scale* as described in Chapter Two? Additionally, the faster our walking speed and the better our balance is in our 40s and 50s, the healthier we are likely to age as well. There's probably a relationship here - the more physically fit we are, the more positive we may feel about our future selves. The right kinds of exercise have a way of lifting our spirits in the present moments as well. We'll develop this further in a later chapter.

So, in the meantime, get your ass moving faster. It's not enough just to walk. You need to walk faster. Oh, and keep your balance while you're doing it.

The BLSA actually provides a hefty dose of hope in changing the perspective on how we age and the findings convincingly suggest that we exert a whole lot of control over how each of us ages. Dr. Luigi Ferrucci, the director of the BLSA, reminds us of the value in this variety of life; *"That's a wonderful thing: it's a window of opportunity. If everyone was on the same deterministic biological trajectory, there would be no hope that we could change it. But the incredible variability shows that the potential to age well is there for everyone. A few people are showing us the way."*

The news about how we age is continuing to improve as other research groups and organizations are reporting similar results as well to what has initially been revealed in the BLSA. Nadia Tuma-Weldon, global director of McCann Worldgroup Truth Central, reported from their *"Truth About Age"* study *"that age is no longer a reliable predictor of just about anything. Age doesn't predict your style, health, aspirations, how you date, or how you behave."* Colin Milner, founder of the International Council on Active Aging, provides additional support - *"The research shows that no two individuals experience aging in exactly the same way or at the same rate. "* And Paul Irving, who chairs the Milken Institute Center for the Future of Aging, reminds us that *"older adults are as diverse and complex and different as any other part of the population, and in many ways more so because their tastes and understandings are refined by a lifetime of experience."*

Are you beginning to see how this traditional view of aging we've held for far too long is a self-fulfilling prophecy that's constructed on a bed of quicksand?

Before leaving this topic of how we age, it's worth taking a moment to review a study by Becca Levy and Martin Slade, colleagues on the faculty at Yale, that's labeled *"Longevity Increased by Positive Self-Perceptions of Aging".* This research found that older individuals who held more positive self-perceptions of aging, measured up to 23 years earlier, lived 7.5 years longer than those with less than positive self-perceptions of aging. Levy and Slade also found that this advantage remained after age, gender, socioeconomic status, social connections, and functional health were included as covariates. Additionally, they learned that healthy aging is partially impacted by a will to live. The sample consisted of 660 individuals aged 50 and older who participated in a community-based survey, the Ohio Longitudinal Study of Aging and Retirement (OLSAR). I make mention of this study because of the relationship between positive self-perceptions of healthy aging more than the reference to an extension of life.

Levy and Slade's findings, by the way, are consistent with the BLSA data referred to moments ago. You'll also learn how our attitudes about aging influence how we experience aging in still another study coming up in a later chapter. As Marty Buccella, an American author, tells us, "*When it comes to staying young, a mind-lift beats a face-lift any day.*"

So the research by Levy and Slade rests in part on the half-empty/half-full glass metaphor and brings to mind for me Norman Cousins' book titled *"The Biology of Hope"* in which he puts forth the belief that positive emotions can enhance the immune system. The dreary outlook is that negative self-perceptions can diminish our lifespan; the bright and sunny one is that positive self-perceptions can prolong it. And then there is the assumption, too, that one's quality of life is enhanced in the present moment - *the here and now* - from positive thoughts about growing older. Sadly, but probably not surprisingly, the opposite looks to be true as well. Dread the passing years and life will simply pass us by while a learned helplessness sets in and we get stuck in the fear of getting older. No thank you. We've already seen enough of this.

Maybe we should consider heeding the words of Carlos Castaneda, the author I discovered in the 1970s, who cautioned that *"we can make ourselves worry or we can make ourselves strong. The amount of effort is the same."* It's a choice we make. It really is. And it's an easy one for me. What about you?

CHAPTER 5

How Our Healthcare System May Help Us Age Prematurely

"America's health care system is neither healthy, caring, nor a system."

Walter Cronkite

IF YOU'RE OLD enough to remember (I know I am), you may recall that Walter Cronkite served as God's spokesperson in the 1960s and 1970s while delivering the nightly news from his heavenly perch in CBS headquarters. Unlike today, where echo chambers exist for virtually any voice we wish to hear, Cronkite's newscast was for One America and he delivered the truth without a political agenda - or so it seemed. So when Walt, deemed the *"most trusted man in America"* at the time, reported that our healthcare system was more akin to a disease care system, he may have been on to something.

Today, a majority of Americans may in many ways agree with Cronkite's assessment of our healthcare system. According to a recent poll from The Associated Press-NORC Center for Public Affairs Research, the poll reveals that public satisfaction with the U.S. healthcare system is dramatically low, with fewer than half of Americans saying healthcare is managed well. Only 12% say it is handled extremely or very well. More precisely, the AP-NORC poll reveals that nearly 8 in 10 admit they are at least moderately concerned about getting access to quality health care when they need it. *"Navigating the American healthcare system is exceedingly frustrating,"* said A. Mark Fendrick, the director of the University of Michigan Center for Value-Based Insurance Design. *"The COVID pandemic has only made it worse."* Frustration looms large as insurance companies provide final approval on most services and treatment plans ...all, critics will say, in the name of profit.

It certainly may be more profitable to deal with disease rather than wellness as modern medicine appears to be shifting towards corporate control. A case in point is Trinity Healthcare of New England recently slapping a lawsuit on Hartford Healthcare for allegedly attempting to monopolize healthcare services in the Greater Hartford, CT area. Another example is Amazon recently moving into healthcare services when it purchased One Medical for $3.9 billion.

This corporate approach reminds me of efforts to monetize public education by creating for-profit grade schools, with proponents arguing they could deliver improved educational services at a lower cost than what local governments are able to provide. Corporate healthcare providers are promising similar results, and they appear to be focusing their efforts on prevention - preserving health - as a means of cutting costs for both patients and providers. In so doing, there is a renewed focus on the primary care practitioner, an otherwise dying breed in the health profession as specialties have been more lucrative practices for doctors in recent years. This is an encouraging development.

I know plenty of physicians and other health care practitioners who abide by the Hippocratic Oath to state confidently that I find this singular focus upon profitability difficult to accept. Likewise, the corporate focus appears to concentrate upon health and not disease. I also understand how frustrating it must be for healthcare practitioners when confronted with the learned helplessness that many of us seem to exhibit these days. *"Fix me, and do it now, please"* is the message we often bring to healthcare practitioners when we suffer from an ailment. Providers today are overwhelmed by an increasingly aging population as well as a spike in health issues caused by factors well within our control...like our body weight.

Still, the healthcare profession can plant self-fulfilling prophecies in the public's mind that may clearly influence behavior, and not the kind we wish for. Here's an example of an unintended message that medical professionals deliver to unsuspecting patients on a fairly regular basis. Below is a promotional announcement - verbatim, no cherry picking - about a workshop recently presented at a local gym by an orthopedic spine specialist;

> *As you grow older, your intervertebral discs begin drying out, wearing away, and shrinking. When this*

happens, you can start experiencing more stiffness and pain in your back. Arthritis, osteoporosis and loss of muscle strength or elasticity may also contribute to pain and back problems.

Join us to learn your options for back pain treatment including when surgery might be beneficial.

Thanks for the heads-up, Doc. Or more accurately, for scaring the bejesus out of me. This surgeon may mean well, but the message is a misleading one. It certainly may be beneficial to warn us of what our backs could become if we just idly sit on our asses waiting for it to happen, but there is no mention of prevention…of what we can do to prevent or at least minimize the inevitable wearing as described in the previous chapter. What can I do in order to *avoid* the maladies mentioned above? Anything? Or do I just bide my time until the pain arrives?

I know first-hand what back pain is. Seven years ago, when I was 65, I had come in from a cold Connecticut winter night in January after a run and decided to check on the condo we were renovating before moving in to it. A box about 12 inches in diameter sat in the middle of the kitchen floor and I attempted to move it elsewhere when I was greeted with paralyzing pain in my lower back and left leg. The box, I discovered afterwards, was filled to the top with kitchen tile slates. Moments later, I found it excruciatingly painful to walk, to move at all. So I didn't. For three days.

I eventually took the next steps, visiting with my primary care physician (PCP) and scheduling an MRI of my lower back.

My PCP then referred me to a back specialist after learning from the MRI that I had arthritis presenting in my facet joints and a mildly herniated disk. The specialist offered surgery as a treatment option. I declined (not easy to do, given the pain I was experiencing). He then suggested an epidural. I declined that, too.

I know too many people who have had back surgery and found only temporary relief, likely because the surgery addressed the symptoms and not the causes. The Mayo Clinic appears to agree - *"Back surgery can help relieve some causes of back pain, but it's rarely necessary. Most back pain resolves on its own within three months."* We just need to be patient... and not choose to become one. As for epidurals, the few I've known to select this option experienced a reduction in symptoms for about six months. And then the pain returned. To be fair, I've heard of others who have felt the pain disappear for more than a few years.

I did my own research and learned that the most effective protection against back pain is a strong core complex. So this is what I set out to do. And I've done it ever since. Core work, previously an afterthought prior to my back injury, is central to every workout I do now. The result has been that my abdominal complex has never been stronger in my life. Believe it or not. It is. I've planked my way to a pain-free back. And this is now my approach with clients who present back pain as a prominent issue to address in training sessions.

As already mentioned, back pain is often symptomatic of issues elsewhere. It's purely speculation on my part, but I do believe that my lower left back issue was the result of the drop foot I previously had on the other side of my body. Because my right leg is still about ten percent weaker than my left leg, I don't produce as much ground force on that leg and, thus, it adversely impacts the strength of my right hip. Guess what - our hips work in conjunction with the opposing quadratus lumborum (QL) (located by each pelvis). So my left QL has had to pick up more of the work and that area of my back likely gave out on me when I pushed too far. I've addressed that muscle imbalance and continue to each passing day.

Anyway, a strong abdominal complex combined with gluteus complex strength as well as quadricep and hamstring strength all in their own ways provide support for my backside. This regimen has also been successful with the clients I've had who have suffered from lower back pain. Warning aside that it takes disciplined, consistent effort on a daily basis to get this protection, core strength has served me so well with my posture, energy level, and disposition that I'm recommending this as the first treatment option in most cases.

My message here is simply one that urges us to examine the services provided. Personally, I've received top-notch care from a wide spectrum of medical professionals - primary care physicians, specialists in their respective fields, nurses, physicians' assistants, physical therapists, massage therapists, acupuncturists. I trust implicitly and comfortably rely upon a small coterie of healthcare professionals I've discovered along the way who attend to my trials and tribulations. In their own way, each has been incredibly helpful with addressing my health issues and otherwise providing caring and compassionate support in my quest to remain active at the level I prefer. It's a partnership I've developed with each. When you find a healthcare practitioner you trust, hold on to her/him. If you're not comfortable with any one of your healthcare support staff, then find another or others you do like and whose professional skills you trust. I tell my family and friends that the *"time to fix a leaky roof is when the sun is shining."* Otherwise, it's too late when the *"rain"* starts falling.

All that said, the medical profession is not omnipotent. Doctors are not infallible. After all, they are human beings with their own biases and flaws. I've received some pretty piss-poor care that was heartless and mindless...for example, one from a cardiologist without a proverbial heart (a single visit was enough before I did my own bypass on him and went elsewhere to find an awesome cardiologist suggested by my PCP) and another with an orthopedic surgeon diagnosing my sore left hip several years ago as a *"51-year-old joint"* (I thanked him for his diagnosis and ended the appointment, but only after letting him know my right hip was 51 at the time as well, and that hip was NOT bothering me). He also advised me to stop running. I still enjoy running, 21 years later. It's probably my favorite exercise to do, albeit a couple times a week.

We need to be giving full attention to our health concerns when visiting with healthcare professionals, and this includes preparing for visits with pertinent questions in hand.

Having said this, the following example is offered for a balanced perspective here. Almost two years ago, I visited with an orthopedic specialist my PCP referred me to in order to learn more about the discomfort in my left knee and to actually verify that it's a torn meniscus and not ligament damage. It was indeed verified and the doctor advised me to continue what I'm doing - strengthening every muscle that supports the knee - because corrective surgery would put me on the *"injured reserve list"* for six months and, even worse, I'd have arthritis in five years from the procedure. He listened to my needs and desires. He understood me. He knew the primary objective was to keep me in play. Cost-benefit? This one was easy for me.

You simply need to recognize when you meet the best in their professions and trust their judgment when counted upon. It doesn't always happen. Or maybe your philosophy runs counter to the healthcare professional's approach. Or whatever. Sometimes a recommendation may not feel right and you need to make sure you don't bite on their *"professional advice"* when they do provide it. Do the necessary follow up. Take responsibility for your own health and well-being, and view your relationship with healthcare professionals as a partnership. Trust is essential. Blind loyalty is not.

Remember - we are products of our decisions and not our circumstances. Had I immediately opted for back surgery seven years ago as a quick solution instead of choosing the admittedly arduous task of strengthening my core, there's no doubt the quality of my life today would be substantially different. That was my decision. I'm so glad I made it.

Modern medicine appears to be drifting towards becoming a triumph of pharmacology. I once had a primary care physician proudly champion the field with this boast - *"we now live in a country where you can get a prescription for just about anything that ails you."* The point was that the solution is in the *"script"*. We already know that solutions are also offered through surgery. *"Scripts"* and surgeries are all-too-common solutions to what hurts us. Sometimes they're necessary. Other times they're not (as noted previously in the Mayo Clinic take on sore backs).

Every decision involves a cost-benefit analysis. Surgery is not free of *"costs"*, nor is any prescription drug. Surgery can address the symptoms but not necessarily the causes (this is not to suggest that surgery doesn't ever address causes - to use a double negative to make my point here. In other words, they do address causes). There is also the potential for disturbances in the area around the surgery - infections forming, nerves damaged around the surgical site and scar tissue forming as well. If not rehabbed properly, range of motion is adversely affected and stiffness sets in, sometimes even permanently. Weigh the costs as well as the benefits.

Drugs, like surgeries, have unintended side effects too. Prescription drugs also interact with other drugs - prescription or over the counter - to produce effects that, when combined, are sometimes worse than what these drugs are designed to treat. Some make us tired. Others bring on dizziness and disorientation, making us more likely to fall. And then there are those that cause weight gain. As for the latter, the five most common medications that cause this unwanted side effect - according to the American Association of Retired People (AARP) - are diabetes drugs, antidepressants, beta blockers (for blood pressure), corticosteroids, and migraine meds. For many, the weight increase can exacerbate the issues that the prescriptions are intended to ameliorate.

"Often, we think of side effects that cause more [physical] symptoms — dizziness, stomach problems, fatigue," says John Batsis, M.D., an associate professor in geriatric medicine and nutrition at the University of North Carolina at Chapel Hill. *"Weight gain, though, can creep up on you."* And for patients who have other medical issues — osteoarthritis or high blood pressure, for example — *"the excess weight can potentially worsen those conditions"*, says Batsis.

Yet research findings point to an increasing number of people consuming drugs that cause weight gain — most notably for conditions that are worsened by added weight, including heart disease and type 2 diabetes. Relying upon data from the 2017-2018 National Health and Nutrition Examination Survey (NHANES), a recent study published in *Obesity* found that one in five U.S. adults take at least one medication that causes weight gain, the most typical being some beta-blockers and diabetes drugs such as insulin and sulfonylureas.

As side effects go, weight gain may not seem like a big deal, especially if treating a life-threatening condition. But in less serious scenarios, added weight can compromise our overall health. People suffering from obesity are at an increased risk for many serious diseases and health conditions, including heart disease, stroke and death, according to the Center for Disease Control and Prevention (CDC). This is no surprise and we'll see why in an upcoming chapter. Even modest weight gain — we're talking 10 to 20 pounds — can have negative health effects. We need to weigh these costs against the benefits derived. Moreover, we need to be better at doing this cost-benefit analysis, and this includes educating ourselves about possible side effects and drug interactions.

Read the fine print and listen closely to the words spoken rapidly on television commercials.

We also need to be better at doing the cost-benefit analysis because it certainly seems like mainstream medicine is leaning towards a healthier life through biochemistry, with less regard for the natural healing powers our internal systems provide and the fact that we have the capability to change our own physiology by means other than drugs (the power of placebos points to this capability, by the way, as conveyed in a beautifully written book titled *"Cure: A Journey Into the Science of Mind Over Body"* by Jo Marchant). This is partly on us - we go to doctors wanting to be fixed. Now. So we seek quick and *"concrete"* solutions in the form of a prescription or surgical procedure and rarely consider our own ability to heal. We often don't take responsibility for our own recovery. Is it a trust issue…we just don't trust our own ability to heal? To do the necessary work?

Critics argue that Big Pharma - a pejorative label, I think - prefers this type of prescription pill treatment and, if you believe the cynics, the hospitals surely love their elective surgeries, too. Although I have already questioned the need for surgery and prescription meds, I don't wish to be cynical here. In all fairness, both Big Pharma and hospitals aid countless people in getting them back on their feet and managing chronic conditions. Thank goodness for antibiotics. And where would we be without the vaccines that eradicate global pandemics? So they profit off of this. Successful businesses - and healthcare is clearly a business - provide quality products that are in demand. Unsuccessful businesses don't. Really, if anyone is to blame, it's us for putting ourselves in these positions that require such costly interventions.

In reality, though, we just might more often be better off if we exercised patience, participated *actively* in our recovery, and allowed our own corrective mechanisms to do their work (Massage therapy, physical therapy, and acupuncture activated self-healing mechanisms in my back treatment as well as with my *"accident"* in January. All are considered healthcare). Better still is managing our health so that we don't need to rely upon the meds. Instead, we numb the pain with medications and, in the process, we lose touch with ourselves. We become comfortably numb, oftentimes unaware this is even happening. And we can suffer unwanted side effects from these medications that further interfere with our ability to engage with life fully as our senses dull and our ability to take in information from our surrounding environments is compromised.

Think about it - we dull our nervous system, the very system designed to help us track our sight, smell, touch, taste, balance (yes - it's a sense), and hearing. We do this all in the name of managing our pain instead of taking the necessary time and making the concerted effort to discover the source of the pain and then fixing that. We choose to feel *nothing* at the expense of including pain among the full range of emotional feelings we could potentially experience otherwise. When our senses lose their effectiveness to monitor our surroundings, we tend to lose our balance in the process.

Even a seemingly benign go-to pill we take when we're trying to manage mild pain can actually be counterproductive. Ibuprofen and other non-steroidal anti-inflammatory drugs (NSAIDs) may, in the long run, extend our pain. Analyzing the health records of 500,000 British adults, researchers discovered that those who used NSAIDs to treat an aching back had a *70 percent* chance of developing *chronic* pain as compared to those who chose alternatives. Supporting evidence comes from studies with mice in which NSAIDs triggered a reduction in neutrophils - white blood cells involved in inflammation. When neutrophils were intentionally blocked by the researchers, it resulted in pain lasting up to ten times longer.

A study involving 98 humans produced similar results - genes linked to inflammation, and specifically neutrophils, were more present and active in those who recovered from pain more quickly. Jeffrey Mogil of McGill University in Montreal, senior author of the study, believes these findings could lead to *"the beginning of the end"* for NSAIDs. *"This class of drugs works in reducing pain early on, but at a great potential cost,"* he reports in the London Times, *"Because if you're unlucky to develop chronic pain, then nothing works very well."*

So can NSAIDs be effective in managing pain? It certainly appears so - when seeking temporary relief. Just be careful about popping them like gummy bears on a frequent basis.

Senior citizens - defined here as anyone 65 or older - are particularly vulnerable to prescription drug abuse and addiction. It's not all that surprising in that this segment of the population has faithfully followed the narrative on aging and we (I'm 72, so therefore the pronoun…) have managed to put ourselves in position for such prescription drugs in order to manage the infirmities we're expected to encounter (reminder: the aforementioned promotional blurb from the spine specialist). This is increasingly becoming an issue among the older population as more ailments become officially classified and more drugs are prescribed as well as advertised through the media to treat these newly discovered infirmities.

According to a report by the Lown Institute, a nonprofit think tank, 42 percent of all older adults in the US take five or more prescription medications a day. Just shy of 20 percent take 10 drugs or more, and over a 20-year period, occurrences of severe drug reactions tripled in this country. Take a look at this comparison of prescription drug consumption from 1994 and again twenty years later as reported by the Lown Institute - *from 1994 to 2014, the percentage of older adults taking five or more prescription meds tripled from 13.8 percent to 42.4 percent.*

This phenomenon has given rise to a new term called poly pharmacy.

And the problem appears to be growing, according to the 2019 report issued by the Institute.

"Over the past few decades, medication use in the US, especially for older people, has gone far beyond necessary poly pharmacy, to the point where millions are overloaded with too many prescriptions and are experiencing significant harm as a result."

Among older individuals, poly pharmacy increases the chance of falls, hospitalization, and other serious medical complications. It's an increasing concern and is expected to worsen as life expectancy lengthens and the aging population increases with it. Us older folks are not only prescribed more drugs but are also at greater risk of severe side effects because our livers tend to be less efficient at metabolizing medications from the bloodstream and then removing them. This risk is compounded by the fact that interactions between some drugs can be unhealthy, even inflicting harmful damage. And, moreover, almost fifty percent of the patients prescribed four or more drugs don't take them as directed, according to a 2020 analysis in the Annual Review of Pharmacology and Toxicology. It's a prescriptive Molotov cocktail, one that actually accelerates our aging.

An aside - according to the CDC, about 80% of COVID deaths accounted for in the past two years have been accompanied by four or more comorbidity factors. But the CDC and health practitioners push only vaccines, face masks, social distancing and lockdowns. There has never been any mention of health management...of how we can lead healthier lives through exercise and proper nutrition. Is this because the CDC doesn't believe that the general population will subscribe to these recommendations and...so why bother? What do you think?

Below is an example of poly pharmacy at work.

When Ann Smith's (changed name) mother, Carol Smith (changed name), was diagnosed with Parkinson's disease in 2010 at the age of 72, she was prescribed a drug called levodopa that she was directed to take four times daily — 7 a.m., 11 a.m., 3 p.m. and 7 p.m. In subsequent years, her doctors prescribed a topical steroid cream for skin issues and prescription drugs for depression, motion sickness, anxiety, acid reflux as well as early-stage breast cancer. That's seven prescriptions, if you're keeping a scorecard. Know anyone like this? I bet you do.

Anyone prescribed multiple medications will surely be challenged to keep track of consumption on a daily basis, and this certainly was the case for Carol. Years later, Carol reported that she really didn't care to take that much medication and felt tied to her home because of the amount of meds she was prescribed. Furthermore, she would sometimes miss doses of her Parkinson's drug, deemed the most important of the drugs prescribed for her. When these forgetful moments would occur, her symptoms of tremors, stiffness and difficulty with speaking and walking would reappear and/or worsen. This resulted in four emergency room visits, two of which required extended hospital stays.

To make the Parkinson's pill (the most critical of all of them) easier to take, Carol's daughter suggested that her mom wean herself off as many meds as she could with her doctor's help. Today she takes only the Parkinson's drug. She reports feeling much better without the other prescription drugs in her system. And Ann says that her mom is far more likely to take levodopa at the correct time now, helping to keep her out of the hospital.

Still another contributing factor to the adverse effects of multiple prescription drugs is the disconnect between a patient's different specialists. Each specialist operates in her/his own orbit of care and may write prescriptions for patients without necessarily knowing what else the patient may be prescribed. This disconnect in communication can give rise to incorrect diagnoses; what may appear to be an illness could instead be the side effect of a different drug. *"All the specialty doctors just focus on their area,"* says Grace Lu-Yao, a cancer epidemiologist at Thomas Jefferson University in Philadelphia. Many patients, including those with cancer that Lu-Yao studies, don't have a doctor who can manage patients and their comprehensive overall treatment. *"Who,"* Lu-Yao says, *"will be the person to look out for potential interactions, or to stop some medication?"*

Carol has a caring daughter. Not everyone has such a caring family member or friend.

There are clearly instances when prescribing multiple medications are necessary. An example may be treating a cardiac patient with cholesterol-reducing statins and blood pressure meds. But when the risks exceed the benefits, then action should be taken and someone needs to intervene on behalf of the patient.

Lu-Yao believes the whole system is dysfunctional. In a recent study, she and her colleagues examined hospitalization rates of prostate, lung and breast cancer patients following chemotherapy treatment. Comparing patients solely on the number of meds prescribed, they found that prostate cancer patients taking five to nine, 10 to 14, and over 15 drugs had respectively 42 percent, 75 percent, and 114 percent higher rates of hospitalization after chemotherapy. Patients with breast and lung cancer had similar results. The researchers emphasized that the group taking more drugs didn't present as being sicker than those taking fewer drugs, according to hospitalization rates in the six months before the chemo treatment. So they concluded that the multiple drugs increased the probability of a hospitalization, and this probability rose with an increasing number of prescriptions.

The Lown Institute estimates that blood thinners, diabetes meds, and opioids account for sixty percent of the emergency room visits caused by adverse drug interactions. The Institute has also identified other drugs that can potentially cause the most harm from adverse side effects - sedative narcotics, over-the-counter meds, blood pressure medication, and antipsychotic drugs.

But for many other elderly patients who are on multiple medications, weaning is not so easy to do. The good news is that many prescribed drugs run their course and are no longer necessary, so these need to be identified by a primary care provider and should be eliminated or replaced with safer medications that are just as effective. The minimal dose effect should be the target. It's estimated that in primary care, about one in five prescriptions given to older adults could be discontinued or changed to a safer alternative. But primary care providers aren't trained in medical schools to de-prescribe meds, only to prescribe them. It's just not in the forefront of their consciousness, although there are efforts under way to address this growing concern.

Pushing for a healthcare system that promotes more judicious drug use and de-prescribing has been an uphill climb. *"Historically, clinical treatment guidelines don't have any recommendations or comment on how or when to stop medications,"* says Emily Reeve, a researcher and pharmacist at the University of South Australia in Adelaide, who has been researching methods to minimize the impact of poly pharmacy in older adults for the past decade. *"How can we make de-prescribing a part of regular practice?"*

Well, here's a dose of good news. Patients appear willing to try. In 2018, a nationally representative survey by Reeve and her colleagues claimed that 92 percent of older adults in the US were willing to stop taking one or more of their medications if their physicians provided stamps of approval. But many doctors lack the formal training to do this correctly. Some general and drug-specific de-prescription guidelines exist, along with websites such as the electronic de-prescribing tool MedSafer that guide doctors and pharmacists through the process — but few of these have been shown to work in clinical practice.

"De-prescribing itself is not a simple action," says Reeve, who is committed to creating de-prescription guidelines that could be used internationally. *"It's not something that can happen within a 10- or a 15-minute appointment."* It involves a thorough review of prescribed drugs, identifying potentially unnecessary or potentially dangerous drugs, securing agreements between doctors and patients to de-prescribe the drugs, and typically a methodical tapering of the medication while the patient is closely monitored.

All that said, some US healthcare facilities are making efforts to address poly pharmacy. One is the Age-Friendly Health Systems program, launched in 2017, in which hospitals and healthcare facilities agree to adhere to the 4Ms — a set of guidelines that guarantees reliable care for the elderly by prioritizing what's most important in their lives, along with their medication, mobility and cognitive abilities. The medication piece involves health care professionals asking if a drug is necessary for the patient, avoiding the use of high-risk medications, creating a plan for safe dose adjustments and de-prescribing when needed.

By the end of 2020, more than 1,950 health care organizations nationwide had linked up with the Age-Friendly Health Systems initiative. Those that incorporated the 4Ms principles reported reduced numbers of hospital readmissions, deaths and cases of delirium. They also reported reductions in health care costs. The goal is to reach a total of 2,600 organizations by June 2023. This sounds like healthcare moving in the right direction and as we should hope to expect.

As much as recent efforts have been launched to improve healthcare services by concentrating more on health and less on disease, there's still a ways to go. If we're to believe the recently retired Director of the National Institutes of Health (NIH), Francis Collins, there's an alarming trend that's unfolding before us. In an interview with PBS, he wondered why it is that there are miraculous medical breakthroughs occurring frequently in our time (i.e., CRISPR technology seems to be real game-changer) while our country concurrently becomes unhealthier? Collins cites data from a 300-page report titled *Shorter Lives, Poorer Health* requested and financed by NIH and conducted by a National Academies of Science, Engineering and Medicine panel. He goes on to say that *"one of the knocks against the National Institutes of Health is that we often seem to be the National Institutes of Disease — that a lot of the focus has been on people who are already diagnosed with some kind of health condition."*

Collins appears to be echoing Cronkite's observation made over fifty years ago, doesn't he?

Well, besides the aforementioned preponderance of drug prescriptions and surgical procedures, we simply need to look around and we'll find an ever-expanding galaxy of healthcare offices and providers surrounding us who are there to treat our mounting infirmities. They seem to be sprouting up everywhere these days, inhabiting space once occupied by store fronts like restaurants, coffee shops, and even business offices. With the modern conveniences of 21st century living now available through our phones for an increasingly older population, there isn't much left for us to do that we can't farm out through some service or app. But can we subcontract our own health and wellness? What does *"wellness"* even mean, anyway? Is it something we can measure?

CHAPTER 6

Measuring Health & Wellness

*The greatest risk to man is not that he aims too high
and misses but that he aims too low and hits.*

Michelangelo

THE US DEPARTMENT of Agriculture has been tracking the entire US food supply since 1950 and in every decade since, including the current one, we've been consuming more fat, more sugar, more meat, and more calories. Plus, we're exercising less. The typical American takes 4,774 steps per day and globally the average is 4,961. The conclusions should be obvious. We're eating more. More of what we're eating are empty calories (processed food). And we're moving less, certainly much less than our ancestors did. All of this, by the way, has become normal. So is it any surprise then that we're a nation experiencing inflation of a different sort than the economic one in which we're currently mired?

Not really. This coincides with Francis Collins' remark made in the previous chapter. It shouldn't surprise us that the effects of this increase in empty calories combined with a concomitant decrease in movement is tipping the scale the wrong way. Weight gain leads to more immobility which leads to more weight gain which leads to more immobility which leads to...a whole host of comorbidities. The surprise, happening in a developed country like the USA, has been that we've come to normalize so much of this unhealthy behavior. This includes our perception of weight.

It turns out that measuring weight has garnered a good deal of attention in recent years. As the nation's collective weight has swelled, so has the percentage of overweight and obese people. But this shouldn't be news to us. We see it all around us. What should become news is the issue of weight in medical offices...whether we're using the right metrics and whether or not patients should be weighed at all.

A typical visit to the doctor usually has us making our way on to a scale as a first step in an exam. We're measured vertically at the same time as well. The two numbers, weight and height, are then combined by dividing the second number into the first to arrive at what's commonly known as body mass index (BMI). Do you know yours?

BMI has been used by medical professionals as a measure of health since the 1980s, with doctors and nurses determining if we're normal weight, underweight, overweight, or obese. The assumptions are that one with a BMI within the normal range is considered healthy and those who fall out of this range are not. It's a pretty simple formula, but it's also a deceptive one in that weight alone doesn't provide a total picture of overall health.

Suzette Pereira is a researcher at Abbott Research and Consulting who studies the role of muscles in health and disease. She tells us that weight by itself doesn't give an accurate portrayal of comprehensive health because it overlooks *"the intricacies of body composition"*– meaning the ratios of muscle, fat, bone, and fluid in our bodies. Still, the BMI guidelines were normalized such that the U.S. Equal Employment Opportunity Commission introduced a regulation in 2015 that would allow businesses to penalize workers up to 30 percent of health insurance costs if their BMIs didn't fall within a certain range. This caused a good deal of blowback among several people, so much so that a team of psychologists at UCLA committed to determining if BMI was a meaningful and accurate measure of overall health.

The psychologists measured subjects' BMIs as well as metabolism and blood pressure. What they learned ultimately challenged the veracity of BMI as a valid and reliable indicator of overall health. Almost half of the people whose BMIs placed them in the overweight or obese category were, in fact, healthy while more than a third of the people with normal BMIs were considered unhealthy. Wait, what - how could this be? It's because the metric of overall weight doesn't differentiate between fat and muscle. With a BMI, a pound of fat is the same as a pound of muscle. If they were indeed the same, then Dwayne "The Rock" Johnson would be obese with a BMI of 34.3 (30 is the "cutoff"). But they're obviously not. There exists a more telling measure - body composition.

Body composition (BC) is a much more accurate depiction of health because it measures lean muscle mass as well as fat. We can infer health and well-being from the amount of muscle on an individual's skeletal frame, with sufficient muscle mass and strength required to live on a day-to-day basis. Knowing how much muscle we're packing and how strong that muscle is can help us determine to what degree - if any - we may be at risk of falling...of moving about at all (1 in 4 adults over the age of 65 will experience a fall-related injury each year). Additionally, as reported by Pereira, muscle mass is directly correlated with recovery from injuries and it also retards the progression of chronic conditions. As we might expect, the greater our muscle mass, the quicker we will recover from injury and the slower chronic illness will seep into our bodies (we'll address this more in Chapter 8). The converse, as expected, is true as well.

We learn in Introduction to Human Anatomy that there are over 600 muscles in our bodies. We don't know much about many of these muscles until we move in such a way as to make them sore. Otherwise, they do their jobs quietly... until they can't do their jobs because we haven't really used them (use it or lose it). In spite of the good intentions we may have, our exercise regimens and routines often falter in the wake of increasing work and family responsibilities. Taking care of ourselves becomes less of a priority. Before we even realize it, weeks and months have passed without us attending to our own physical needs.

So this unintentional neglect eventually leads to muscles weakening and we begin to feel less fit. This is where the traditional narrative helps us to understand why we feel this way - of course, we're getting old. After the age of 40, we're told, we can lose up to 8 percent of our muscle mass each decade. After we turn 70, we can double that loss, up to 15 percent a decade - **unless we do something about it...** like performing exercises that use these muscles. It's pretty simple. And it works. Exercise is a medicine. A really effective and inexpensive one. But we have to do it consistently to feel its effects. This is not so simple. More on this will come in later chapters.

The most critical step we can take in maintaining our lean muscle mass health requires us to pay attention - to listen to our bodies. It doesn't require us to do math calculations to arrive at our BC. Pereira advises, *"If you know the signs of muscle loss, the biggest thing is you feel it before you can actually measure it."* As we've seen, BC is definitely more accurate than BMI.

That said, it's still a metric, and it's on each of us to make sense of the number by regularly asking ourselves if we *"feel"* different...if we notice changes in our day-to-day routine. *"We are working on more tools to measure lean body mass, but that comes with education too,"* says Pereira. *"Once you know that you have low muscle mass, then you know what you need to do to intervene. It's never too late."* We can benefit at any age...if we just find a way to do it.

If you're interested in calculating your BC, it's fairly simple to do. First weigh yourself on a body fat scale (there are plenty of home versions) to determine how much body fat you're carrying. Then simply subtract your body fat weight from your total weight and you'll arrive at your lean muscle mass weight. For example, let's say Sally is 150 pounds and her body fat percentage is 20 percent. Sally would subtract 30 from 150 to arrive at 120 pounds of lean skeletal muscle mass, internal organs, and bones. Will you take this?

As we've seen with *"The Rock"*, body fat percentage is often confused with BMI. They are entirely different measures. A BMI of 25 is not the same as a body fat percentage rate of 25 - the latter being the line of demarcation on classifying someone as *"overweight"*. Let's return for a moment to Sally and add her 150 pound friend, Sarah, for comparison sake. Sarah, by the way, is the same height as Sally. We already know Sally has 20 percent body fat, leaving her with 120 pounds of lean muscle mass. Sarah, on the other hand, has a body fat percentage of 30. What's this mean? It translates into Sarah possessing 105 pounds of lean muscle mass, organs, and skeletal bones, with the rest being subcutaneous fat. See a difference? Same BMI. Much different BC.

We haven't even addressed the significance of where the body fat is located (around the belly is the worst place). But, clearly, this example should reveal the inaccuracy of BMI as a measure of health. It's a metric that may be convenient for medical practitioners to use, particularly because it's noninvasive (although some doctors' offices are now skipping the weigh-in if deemed to be too sensitive for the patient), but we can clearly see its flaws.

Other measures typically taken in doctors' offices are heart rate, respiratory rate, blood pressure, and body temperature. Although these numbers may be important, even critical in emergency-care situations, they fluctuate within a range that otherwise don't provide us with a realistic sense of how functionally fit and durable we may be in the face of our day-to-day challenges and eventual decay. There's a difference between health and wellness, with the former seen as the absence of disease. The Global Wellness Institute defines wellness as *"the active pursuit of activities, choices and life-styles that lead to a state of holistic health."* Other metrics actually may be much more telling for measuring our level of wellness.

Walking speed is one such metric. Of course, this is the go-to exercise for many and the most often recommended by medical practitioners. Some even add the word *"brisk"* to it, although brisk often goes undefined. In a study of approximately 35,000 people aged 65 years or older published in the *Journal of the American Medical Association*, those who strode at about 2.6 feet per second over a short distance—which would amount to a mile in about 33 minutes, not even close to a brisk pace—were likely to reach their average life expectancy. With each speed spike of around 4 inches per second, the chance of dying in the next decade fell by about 12 percent. (Not coincidentally, stride length - how long each step is that we take - has been shown to correlate positively with cognitive clarity. Shorter strides that morph into shuffling can be indicative of cognitive decline. Less physical activity results in less blood flow to the brain).

You may recall that walking speed was addressed several pages back, with the caution that it's not enough to simply walk. Pace is critically important. Several studies have proven this to be the case. We'll address walking speed in greater detail later on here.

Still other measures exist that may be more accurate predictors of functional fitness and longevity. In 2018, a study published by BMI (not to be confused with body mass index), a group that conducts research on medical issues, that included over half a million middle-aged people discovered that lung cancer, heart disease, and all-cause mortality were accurately predicted by the strength of a person's grip. That's right. How hard you squeeze my hand when you shake it can predict for me (and you) how many years you have remaining in this life. Wonder why we haven't seen store fronts popping up with certified *"handshake readers"*.

Other prior studies have produced similar results. A study reported in <u>sciencenorway.no</u> of over 6800 Norwegians between the ages of 50 and 80 measured grip strength by pressing a rubber ball and learned that, among those in their eighties, it was a valid and reliable predictor of individuals in this subset of making it to the century mark.

Another group of scientists working with the Honolulu Heart Program and the Honolulu-Asia Aging Study proposed a simple way to measure disability and longevity in human beings. Between 1965 and 1970, they evaluated about 8,000 healthy men with an average age of 54. Each subject was evaluated for his maximal handgrip strength and were examined for conventional risk factors as well. The scientists followed the men for an average of 25 years with regular checkups. In that span of time, 37% of the men perished. Those who survived were from 71 to 93 years-old. Their primary conclusion from the study was that grip strength in midlife was not a predictor for longevity but it did correlate with disability. The men who exhibited the greatest grip strength in middle age, even after chronic illnesses were taken into account, had the lowest risk of disabilities and dependency in old age.

Still another study, this one with a large sample size, was published online June 23, 2022, by *JAMA Network Open* and it reported that poor handgrip strength in midlife was associated with cognitive decline ten years later. More than 190,000 dementia-free men and women (average age 56) were involved in the study and followed for at least 10 years. Participants took tests that measured handgrip strength, problem-solving skills, memory, and reasoning abilities, and also underwent brain imaging. Comparing people who had higher handgrip strength scores at the start of the study with subjects' lower grip scores, the latter were more likely to later have problems with thinking and memory, brain imaging markers of vascular dementia, and diagnoses of dementia.

If you're still not impressed, then consider another study in Sweden involving handgrip with 18-year-olds in the Swedish military that provided sufficient information to predict cardiovascular disease 25 years later. Of note - it seems like age doesn't matter with the accuracy of this metric. You can be 80 or 18. How about that - your hand grip can reveal your grip on life. Just by knowing how hard you can squeeze a ball will predict how many years you have left to "*play*".

So grab a rubber ball while you're walking and double your pleasure!

Still not convinced? OK. Then let's look at another study that raised eyebrows recently for claiming that our ability to complete push-ups could actually predict the onset of heart disease. Stefanos Kales, a professor at Harvard Medical School, had the bright idea that the leading cause of death of firefighters while in the line of duty wasn't sucking in smoke or getting burned but sudden cardiac arrest. Smoke typically doesn't cause cardiac arrest, nor do skin burns. Heart attacks, Kales figured, are usually triggered by coronary artery disease. So even in a high-risk profession like firefighting, firefighters are most likely to die of the same thing as everyone else - heart disease. Kales arranged a study to determine if this was, in fact, the case.

This longitudinal cohort study of 1104 active adult firemen, reported in the JAMA, found a significant **negative** correlation between baseline push-up capacity and cases of cardiovascular disease risk across 10 years of follow-up. The male firefighters who were able to complete more than 40 push-ups had far fewer cardiac episodes and exhibited lower rates of cardiovascular disease when compared with those completing fewer than 10 push-ups. Pushups and heart health - who would have ever thought?

Kales learned that pushup strength was an even more accurate predictor of cardiovascular disease than a traditional sub maximal treadmill test. *"The results show a strong association between push-up capacity and decreased risk of subsequent cardiovascular disease,"* Kales reports. *"Before the American Disabilities Act, a fire or police department might have a BMI standard where they won't accept you,"* Kales says. *"Now they want functional standards."* They want to know if you can put out fires and not what your waist size is. It's also a simpler and much less expensive way to measure heart health.

Here's the thing, though. We need to be careful about mixing correlation with causation as we first reminded ourselves back in Chapter Two with the study referencing the *National Poll On Healthy Aging.* That said, relationships do exist, with cause and effect inferred. These research findings can spread to the general population so that more may reap the benefits. The push-up study could easily be applied to individuals beyond firefighters. *"Push-ups are another marker in a consistent story about whole-body exercise capacity and mortality,"* claims Michael Joyner, a researcher at the Mayo Clinic who concentrates his efforts on researching the limits of human performance. *"Any form of whole-body engagement becomes predictive of mortality if the population is large enough."* Gather enough people, find commonalities and consistencies in whole-body behavior among them, and you can begin to tell the future on those behaviors.

So what's all this mean? Well, it doesn't mean that our health and wellness can be summed up **solely** by the number of pushups we can perform or how strong our handshakes are or even how fast we can walk. There's no need to worry that your doctor will be ordering you anytime soon to get down on the floor and *"give me ten pushups"* instead of stepping on the scale. What it does say, though, is Kales concluded that firefighters who could bang out more pushups probably had low blood pressure, cholesterol, triglycerides, and blood sugar, and they likely didn't smoke. Those with limp handshakes and weak grip strength were more likely to practice unhealthy behaviors - smoking cigarettes, eating fewer fruits and vegetables and more processed foods, - that resulted in higher weight and body fat percentages. And weak muscles. As for walking, we've seen that faster is so much better. These inferences, by the way, are all lifestyle habits - both good and bad.

Most experts estimate that the number of people among us in the USA who can do a single, legitimate push-up is likely somewhere between 20 or 30 percent. Not very impressive, is it? But that's not the result of aging and decay. It's more likely because of inactivity. We lose it because we don't use it. Or we never get it because we don't ever develop it. It's often that simple. *"Most people could get to the point of doing 30 or 40—unless they have a shoulder problem or are really obese,"* Joyner says.

Most of us could…if we wanted to…and we did the smart work to get there. Most of us could also walk faster. And we've seen how all of this could potentially help us grow older in healthier ways.

But do we sell ourselves short as we age? Do we underestimate what we can do because we're faithfully following the script on aging? Was Janis Joplin right when she said *"You are what you settle for?"* Or Michelangelo, who warned us about aiming too low? Do we just say *"screw it"* and give up? I think some of us do. If you're one of these, I hope you're still here. The rest of this book is especially for you.

CHAPTER 7

How Old Are You Really?

"How old would you be if you didn't know how old you are?"

Satchel Paige

A DIFFERENT KIND of math has been taking hold in recent years that you likely recognize and may even have adopted. Seventy is the new 50, 60 the new 40. What's going on? Can we just be any age we decide to be? Is there an element of truth to this?

Let's take a moment and return to that room with all the 65 year-old people in it that we considered back in Chapter 5. You know - the one that's adjacent to the room with the 21-year-olds. Recall that we learned the older group was more diverse in its makeup than the youngsters - that there were likely 65 versions of what it means to be 65 years-old, according to the BLSA study. So who in the room among those senior citizens would be considered the "youngest"? The "oldest"? Who could legitimately identify as a "45 year-old" (using the unofficial equation of chronological age minus 20)? How would we know? How *could* we know? What would we measure? Is this even possible?

Well, a growing group of scientists that studies aging believes it's definitely possible. These same scientists believe that chronological age (CA) is different from biological age (BA), and that it's the latter to which we need to turn our attention because it's the latter that's much more telling than CA by itself. Sounds promising. But how? They claim to be able to identify biomarkers in individuals that they can then use to accurately measure biological age. After all, this is how the BSLA study is being conducted - researchers are doing blood work, physical tests for mobility, cognitive testing, and body composition on its participants. Even more, these scientists contend that they can identify the variables that influence aging and, in the process, hope to slow the progress of chronic disease and allow us to possibly live longer. It's pretty lofty stuff.

It's actually pie-in-the-sky lofty fluff, according to another group of scientists who aren't so convinced. These skeptics think their misguided colleagues are selling snake oil to similarly misguided and gullible senior citizens. Who's right? Besides, even if it is possible, do I really want to know my biological age? What good would it do me?

An aside - if you're struggling with this notion of an "age" other than the chronological number we're accustomed to, the reality is we've already been dealing with another kind of number related to our chronological age most all of our lives - IQ, or intelligence quotient. Your IQ is calculated by taking a score you earn on an *"intelligent test"*, dividing it by your chronological age, and multiplying it by 100. For example, if your score is equivalent to what is *"expected"* of a ten year-old and you're 10 years old, your IQ equals 100 - positioned perfectly in the middle of the average range. If you earn this same score on that same measure and you're eight years old, you're a smart little ass with an IQ of 125. Of course, IQ tests have been the subject of intense debate in recent decades as some critics argue these tests are culturally biased and others believe they only measure a narrow slice of intelligence. Either way, we seem to have accepted this measure of age.

You can probably figure out what biological age means as compared to the raw number (chronological age), but let's differentiate it here for the sake of clarity. It's a measure of health that can be more or less than your chronological age, and this measure can help us understand our own health moving forward much more accurately than chronological age is able to do (recall several pages back with mention of how we age in +/- increments of one per year). Proponents of this theory determine BA with biomarkers measured for each individual based on the belief that our organs and cells age in different ways as compared to our CA. David Sinclair of the Harvard Medical School refers to this BA as a *"credit score for your body."*

Let's return to the question - *"So what's in it for me?"* Well, if you know your BA and you're not thrilled with it, you can do something about it. You can change your lifestyle and do all the stuff already mentioned here that's good for you. This is the claim of the BA proponents. They also believe that knowing your BA can help you predict how many more years you have remaining to play.

Of course, if you too think this is pie-in-the-sky lofty fluff, then none of this matters. It may be good enough for you to gauge how old you are simply by how old you feel. Or you may just simply go with the digits already assigned to you. As for lifestyle changes, what's the point in changing anything if it really has no effect on your way to eventual obsolescence? It's all up to the genes, anyway. This is the position assumed by the skeptics, although my sense is that their issue has more to do with extending the lifespan - it's not happening, no matter what - than any specific measure of a biological age.

I don't know about you, but I'd like at least some degree of control over my pace towards the checkout counter. After all, there is substantial evidence that the environment plays a role in a human being's development over time. This evidence is observed in longitudinal studies involving identical twins raised in separate environments. That they can age in different ways - sometimes with dramatic differences - strongly suggests the influence of external factors in the aging process. Nurture appears to be just as important - and maybe even more so - than nature. Recall the Epigenetics Theory of Aging?

So I hope you're still listening, but you likely want to know specifically what they're measuring in you. What are these biomarkers? And where are they?

Steve Horvath believes he knows what they are and where to find them. You may recall seeing his name mentioned in Chapter 3 when we briefly examined the epigenetic theory. Horvath is a professor at UCLA and his claim to fame is developing the Horvath aging clock which he promotes as a highly accurate molecular biomarker of aging. This UCLA Bruin is selling the promise that he can identify your BA within a range of five years and predict how long you're likely to continue lapping the sun going forward.

Horvath's crystal ball is an **epigenetic clock** and it utilizes a biochemical test to measure age. You likely need a Ph.D. in biochemistry (and probably that eight-year old's IQ of 125) to grasp the details of this test and explain the processes involved. I don't have one, but I've relied on others who do and we'll see if we can translate this into sensible terms.

Recall from Chapter 3 that epigenomes regulate DNA by signaling on and off mechanisms (*the epigenetic theory*) like a switchboard operator. Horvath's biochemical test is based on DNA methylation levels that are related to the aforementioned epigenomes. By comparing DNA methylation age (estimated age) to chronological age, Horvath and associates can identify measures of age acceleration - or at what speed we're traveling through this life (slower, in this case, is better…much better). Age acceleration is measured as the difference between DNA methylation age and chronological age. This is likely why we see some people appearing to be an age other than the one by which they identify (the chronological number, right?), whether this is older or younger - plus or minus a few years. It's their DNA methylation age they're showing!

Methylation can alter the behavior of a DNA segment without changing the gene sequence measuring the accumulation of methyl groups to one's DNA molecules. So this is where we see genes not only controlling behavior but these same genes are also being controlled by one's epigenomes.

Let's look at it another way. Think for a moment that a chromosome is the magnetic tape of a cassette (another outdated reference, but it works here and has elsewhere as well) and each gene is compatible to a track recorded on the tape. Epigenetics are pieces of adjustable adhesive tape that will cover or reveal specific tracks, essentially rendering them unreadable or readable. So there are methylating agents that block gene expression and there are other molecules, called acetyl groups, that have the effect of exciting gene expression. Note that gene sequences are not altered in this process. They are simply turned on or off.

Let's return to Horvath's clock. His "Big Ben" is described as a method of age estimation that relies upon 353 epigenetic markers on the DNA. These markers are said to measure the DNA methylation of CpG dinucleotides. Since age has been found to have a strong effect on DNA methylation levels at tens of thousands of CpG sites, Horvath and *"friends"* can describe a highly accurate DNA methylation age in human beings.

Horvath's finding that the DNA methylation age of blood accurately predicts all-cause mortality in later life even after adjusting for known risk factors is consistent with a variety of causal relationships. Similarly, measures of physical and mental fitness are associated with the epigenetic clock (lower abilities are related to age acceleration).

What's particularly impressive about Horvath's epigenetic clock is its applicability to a wide range of tissues and cell types. The clock is accurate across *"time zones"*, or various tissues. Because it's possible to contrast the ages of different tissues from the same subject, the clock can be used to identify tissues that exhibit evidence of accelerated age due to disease.

It's worth revisiting those twin studies once more to highlight the influence of our environments upon gene expression and to reiterate the level of control we seem to exert over this expression. We've already observed how our environment influences our genome through epigenetic modifications. It's conceivable, in monozygotic (identical) twin pairs, to identify sizable differences in their respective lives. One could become overweight and the other could remain thin; one could develop a host of infirmities and the other could be a picture of perfect health. How can this be if they inherited the same set of genes from the same egg? It has to be the influence of environmental factors on each twin's epigenomes. What else could it be?

Horvath and like-minded researchers argue that it's the epigenetic changes that are triggered by the environment that produce these noticeable differences. Our cells regularly take in all kinds of stimuli informing them (the cells) about its environment, so that it adapts its activity to the situation. These signals, including those *related to our lifestyles* (diet, exercise, smoking, stress), can bring about changes in the expression of our genes - both good and bad - without changing their sequence.

If this is, in fact, all true and not pie-in-the-sky fluff, then we need to examine more closely the behaviors that we can integrate into our lives that will slow down the second hand on Horvath's clock; that is, if you wish to slow this time lapse. Those residing in the naysayers' camp subscribe to the belief that little, if anything, can be done to extend life. It is what it is, as they say, and it's already programmed into us. *Let me reiterate - this book is NOT about stretching out our life span...it's specifically about extending our health span.* Note that the average health span in the US is 66 years and this currently still leaves us, on average, with at least a decade of life in ill health. Why would we want to extend this period of sickness for another decade? Why - unless we change the narrative.

Maybe it would be useful for us to know where we are along this continuum of life so that we may introduce lifestyle changes that can slow the pace of age acceleration if we wish to take at least some control of this process. *If this is your wish , then exercise - specifically strength training - may be one such behavior that you should consider more seriously.* You may be saying - *"Well, I'm already doing this."* OK. Let's see. We'll return to this topic of muscles in the next chapter and to a more comprehensive explanation in later chapters. But before we do so, it's worth looking at other *"markers"* of aging that have been identified and that may be associated with the pace at which we are marching through life.

Another such marker is something you may have already heard of - they're called telemeres, and they are a recent discovery that provides even more evidence that our lifestyles exert a significant influence on our trip through this experience of life. The 2009 Nobel Prize in Medicine was awarded to American researchers Elizabeth Blackburn, Carol Greider, and Jack Szostak *"for solving a major biological problem"* that was cast as a question - how can chromosomes be replicated wholly during cell division and how are they protected from destruction or debasement over a duration of time? These Nobel laureates have provided compelling evidence that the solution to this problem is at the ends of the chromosomes - fragments of human DNA called "**telomeres**" that were discovered by Szostak - and in the enzyme that forms them - "**telomerase**" found by Blackburn and Greider. Blackburn has also proven that the length of telomeres and the behavior of the telomerase enzyme are critical factors in other diseases (chronic inflammatory diseases - addressed in a moment) and aging.

So we know that telomerase is an enzyme that controls the length of the *"telomeres"*, which are repeated segments of non-coding DNA positioned at the end of each chromosome. These telomeres are often described as kind of like the small plastic pieces that protect the tips of our shoelaces and are called *"aglets"*. They form small covers at the ends of the chromosomes, preventing the genetic material from fraying and are the aglets that tend to shorten over time... another way of saying *"as we age"*. Thus, telomerase has the capacity to influence telomeres, effectively shortening and/or lengthening them. The length of our telomeres can reveal how *"old"* we may be - longer telomeres are better. And we can see through this that aging is a dynamic process that can be accelerated or delayed. It seems like we have the capability to step on the gas pedal AND apply the brakes with our telomeres, and *how* we choose to live in our own personal worlds may have more of an impact upon this stop-go mechanism than previously thought.

The research conducted by Blackburn and her team have contributed significantly to the theory that the inordinate shortening of the telomeres marks the descent into the senescence of cells, and this shortening increases the risks of degenerative diseases, cancers, cardiovascular diseases and the like. It appears that our in-built monitoring system recognizes these senescent cells as dangerous threats and, in response, releases pro-inflammatory substances (free radicals or cytokines - you heard about the latter with "cytokine storms" erupting in Covid patients who had multiple comorbidities) which cause pain and chronic pathologies that show up as we age and which *we automatically attribute to aging rather than our lifestyle choices.*

Blackburn and Greider proposed the hypothesis that individuals age at different rates because of complex interactions between their genes. They explain that one's emotional relationships, social environment, lifestyle, personal stressors and, in particular, the way all of these interact with each other are contributing factors to this process. From this, Blackburn and Greider concluded that the telomeres could stop shortening and even lengthen due to the influence of the telomerase enzyme. Aging is, thus, a dynamic process that could be sped up or slowed down.

Another small study conducted by scientists at UC San Francisco and the Preventive Medicine Research Institute, a nonprofit public research institute in Sausalito, Calif. that investigates the effect of diet and lifestyle choices on health and disease, reports that *changes in diet, exercise, stress management and social support may result in longer telomeres.* Published online on Sept. 16, 2013 in The Lancet Oncology, the researchers followed for five years thirty-five males with early-stage prostate cancer to investigate the relationship between comprehensive lifestyle changes and both telomere length and telomerase activity. All the men were closely monitored through screening and biopsies. Ten of the subjects engaged in lifestyle changes that included a plant-based diet (high in fruits, vegetables and unrefined grains, and low in fat and refined carbohydrates), moderate exercise (walking 30 minutes a day, six days a week), and stress reduction (gentle yoga-based stretching, breathing, meditation). They also participated in weekly group support. These males were then compared to the twenty-five subjects who were not asked to make major lifestyle changes.

The group that made the lifestyle changes experienced a *"significant"* increase in telomere length of approximately ten percent. Moreover, a positive correlation emerged such that the more participants changed their behavior by adhering to the recommended lifestyle program, the more significant their improvements were in telomere length. Note that telomeres typically shorten as we age. By comparison, the males in the control group who didn't adjust their lifestyles had measurably shorter telomeres – nearly 3 percent shorter – when the five-year study ended.

The researchers suggest that these the findings may not be limited to men with prostate cancer and likely can be both relevant and applied to the general population. *"We looked at telomeres in the participants' blood, not their prostate tissue,"* said Dean Ornish, MD, UCSF clinical professor of medicine, and founder and president of the Preventive Medicine Research Institute. *"So often people think 'Oh, I have bad* genes, there's nothing I can do about it,'" Ornish said. "But these findings indicate that telomeres may lengthen to the degree that people change how they live. Research indicates that longer telomeres are associated with fewer illnesses and longer life."

If true, this is pretty remarkable. Is there a reason why we shouldn't believe this? Why we wouldn't want to believe it?

One more marker we'll consider before leaving this chapter was briefly touched upon moments ago. It's inflammation, and there are two kinds. One is our ally and the other an enemy. Our lifestyle choices may be contributing to the latter, igniting perpetual, low-level brush fires within us that lead to chronic illness and disease.

Inflammation is a critical function of our factory-installed immune system that's triggered instantly when it senses an intrusive pathogen or damaged tissue. Think of a sprain when you turn your ankle or a bruise when you get hit by an object - swelling occurs around the site of the injury as blood rushes to begin the repair process. This is our immune system at work, automatically performing its role of healing and repairing damaged tissue. A spike in body temperature that we call a fever is another such example when a virus invades us and makes us ill.

Acute inflammation occurs immediately upon injury or illness and it typically lasts a few days. Cytokines and chemokines promote the movement of neutrophils and macrophages to the site of the injury and related inflammation. Pathogens, bruises, toxins, burns, and frostbite are some of the regular causes of acute inflammation. I'm sure you're familiar with most all of these invaders. A healthy immune system that's functioning properly will typically do its work in a few days to a week or so and will *"leave"* the injured area when the invading substances have been neutralized. Be cautious with anti-inflammatory meds here as noted in a previous chapter with NSAIDs.

Some injuries heal more quickly than others. Injured sites that are more complex - like our organs and glands - take more time to heal. Those less complicated, like skin, heal more quickly. If it's not possible to grow tissue at the injured site, scar tissue will form to fill in empty spaces. An important point to note is that the amount of inflammation arising at the injured site needs to be the right amount - too little and the invaders remain; too much and a cytokine storm erupts that causes a whole lot of collateral damage that can lead to metabolic issues. This latter type is called chronic inflammation and it's the kind that causes internal climate change. When this occurs, trouble begins to heat up and cytokine storms begin swirling internally.

Chronic inflammation is quite different from the acute kind referred to above. If the injury remains and the immune response is constantly called upon to react, or if we have a condition that is causing the immune system to respond *as if* there is a threat, then the natural inflammatory response can continue and cause harm to the body instead of healing it. The harm we're talking about includes rheumatoid arthritis, cancer, cardiovascular disease, diabetes, asthma, hepatitis C, autoimmune diseases, and quite possibly Alzheimer's disease. It's why Maria Borelius, a biologist and author of *Health*

Revolution: Finding Happiness and Health Through an Anti-Inflammatory Lifestyle refers to chronic inflammation as a *"gateway to disease."* As we can see, these low-level brush fires that continue unabated can eventually lead to sprawling forest fires recognized as debilitating metabolic disease conditions. Just as troubling is that all of this happens *"quietly"* - we think we're just fine on the *"outside"* while we're burning up on the inside. We're feeling just fine...until suddenly we're not. Borelius describes it this way - *"It's like if you have a village with a fire brigade and there are constant small fires they're constantly trying to put out; they won't have any power when something big comes along,"* It's kind of like we're fried at that point...pun intended.

Many of us older people develop a condition called inflammaging, and this is characterized by increased levels of blood inflammatory markers that correlate very positively to chronic morbidity, disability, frailty, and premature death. Note here that inflammaging isn't so much a consequence of aging as much as it is one of lifestyle choices. It's possible for some of us to be genetically susceptible to chronic inflammation. Other more likely contributing factors are excessive weight, obesity, increased gut permeability, cellular senescence (we've already seen this), oxidative stress caused by dysfunctional mitochondria (addressed in the next chapter), and chronic infections.

Let's make mention of a few critical points related to chronic inflammation and inflammaging. Elevated levels of pro-inflammatory markers in the blood and other tissues have been found to be predictive of cardiovascular diseases, frailty, multiple comorbidities, and a decline in cognitive and physical functioning. With individuals who are overweight, and especially those who are obese, visceral fat (particularly around the midsection where several of our organs are located) generates pro-inflammatory chemicals and is *"invaded"* by macrophages, lymphocytes, and senescent cells with a senescence-related phenotype that contributes to inflammaging. None of this is anything we should long for. For this we should be certain.

It's all pretty dangerous stuff that raises two important questions - Can we get tested for this? And, if so, should we? After all, it's quite possible that we could have elevated levels of inflammation and not know it, particularly with those among us who are obese and, thus, potentially diabetic or who may be suffering from cardiovascular disease. So wouldn't it make sense to measure levels so that we could adjust our lifestyles in response and reduce the amount we're carrying?

It certainly would seem so…in the right circumstances. And there are medical tests currently available to determine the prevalence of inflammation, but these measures don't distinguish between the acute and chronic kinds. One of the more common tests for inflammation is C-reactive protein (CRP) and this identifies the level of inflammation in one's liver. It's often used to evaluate one's risk of cardiovascular disease, but systemic (full body) inflammation can make CRP rise to 100 mg/L or more and may trigger other metabolic diseases as well. CRP is also helpful in monitoring levels of inflammation for those suffering from rheumatoid arthritis.

Still, should we test for inflammation in the abstract or instead evaluate for specific infirmities that produce such inflammation? Robert H. Shmerling, MD, Senior Faculty Editor at Harvard Health Publishing answers the question this way - *"By looking for evidence of inflammation through a blood test without any sense of why it might be there is much less helpful than having routine healthcare that screens for common causes of silent inflammation, including excess weight, diabetes, cardiovascular disease, hepatitis C as well as other chronic infections, and autoimmune disease."* Who needs one more wasteful test? This is the thinking here with regard to inflammation. Critics of these tests for inflammation claim that those who support them are companies who produce and market them.

Having said this, we shouldn't disregard the possible presence of chronic inflammation because, as we've seen, it can wreak havoc internally. Instead, know that excess weight may be a harbinger for the silent assassin lurking in our systems. When excess weight is an issue (body fat percentage in excess of 25% for males and 30% for women), then it may be a wise move to test for diabetes and other related potential ailments as a starting point. If a fire is burning, it makes sense to control it before the flames spread uncontrollably into a category one cytokine storm. An ounce of prevention is worth the avoidance of a scorched immune system.

So, here we are. With all of the research findings - biological clocks, telomeres, inflammation - related to measures of how we age, it begs two questions: *"How old am I really?"* And *"Is it possible for me to slow this train and even reverse course?"*

What do you think? The evidence as presented here and in previous chapters certainly supports the real possibility. Whatever the case and wherever you stand, I wonder if we should forget our chronological age and just live according to how we feel. In the end, it's the feeling of youthfulness that we may hope to retain (or recapture) as we grow older, isn't it? After all, how old would you be if you didn't know how old you are?

This is really all about energy and how much we have at our disposal. It's there. There just seems to be less of it available as we age. But, paradoxically, it is less the consequence of aging than it is our lifestyles. Lifestyle choices, as we've seen repeatedly in previous pages, are sapping us. We need to find this energy within us. The secret is in the source, and the source of this raw energy may very well be found in our muscles…when they're used as they're meant to be used.

CHAPTER 8

Muscle Matters

*"We don't stop exercising because we grow old – we
grow old because we stop exercising."*

Dr. Ken Cooper

IT TURNS OUT that muscle matters more to us than we think.
Without muscle, of course, we wouldn't be able to move from
one location to another, pick up and put down objects, even
pick up and put down our own bodies, never mind that we
wouldn't be able to breathe or perform other natural functions, either. We often only notice our muscles when they're
sore, and it's rarely pleasant when we have such experiences.
We often notice, too, that we may tend to lose our muscle
strength as we get older. If this is the case, the effects of muscle loss are multiple and affect us in ways that go beyond
simply moving our own bodies or lugging around objects.
**We need to use our muscles so that they're able to execute
the cellular functions required for us to remain healthy, well-
balanced human beings.** It's that important and I hope you'll
see why in the next several pages.

Let's begin this with a closer look at the kinds of muscle we have in our possession. There are generally three kinds - smooth muscles are of the involuntary type and are controlled by our autonomic nervous system (i.e., muscles in our intestinal walls and arterial walls), cardiac muscle that pumps blood (our hearts), and skeletal muscle that attaches to our skeletal systems and helps us move about. It's the latter group that we seem to be most familiar with and the one that requires us to *voluntarily* use them. These muscles, as you will soon see, are also involved in vital metabolic processes.

Skeletal muscle is the most extensive single tissue type in the human body. We come equipped with more than 640 muscles that comprise between 30 and 40 percent of our total body weight (recall the difference between BMI and body composition from the previous chapter). I wish to emphasize here that skeletal muscle burns about *twenty-five percent* of our body's energy at rest. Fat, on the other hand, burns *zero percent* (So here's another "perk" for having more muscle mass...you can *"spend"* calories while sitting still).

When we think of well-developed skeletal muscles, bodybuilders come to mind as do elite-level athletes. Of course, we can also observe perfectly chiseled musculature on the Ancient Greek and Roman sculptures and portraits posing for us in museums everywhere around us. In fact, we can slip back even further in time to several thousand years ago when our really ancient, muscle-strapping ancestors were spending their days in perpetual movement. There were no UberEats or Amazon Delivery back then. They were searching for whole foods on their own to deliver back to their campsites. Our ancestors were tireless exercise machines as evolutionary processes made sure that the strong survived in order for them to hunt and gather with any degree of success. In many ways, we have our ancestors to blame for the ill effects that a sedentary, twenty-first century lifestyle is bringing us today. How?

Evolution has brought forward for us modern-day humans several of the metabolic traits of our hunter-gatherer ancestors that formed out of the need to fuel their daily physical demands. Research by Frank W. Booth and P. Darrell Neufer that appeared in *American Scientist* strongly suggests that these metabolic processes require us to continue moving, and the fact that we're not moving is undoubtedly contributing to the mounting health issues confronting many people today. Our inattention to the 600+ skeletal muscles attached to our body frames may very well be a major contributing factor in the spike of chronic diseases that now cause the bulk of today's deaths. With this being the case, it would appear then that muscular development and strength aren't just for the Greek and Roman gods or today's elite athletes. Muscular strength is necessary for us all if we wish to avoid the chronic diseases that compromise the quality of life before ultimately doing us in for good. It puts *"use it or lose it"* in another realm and on another level.

You may not like me referring to us as *"plastic"* people. But we are. We are in this sense - skeletal muscle is continually shaped in its composition to meet the specific or repeated demands placed on it. This is a process called *plasticity,* and this is what makes us plastic. Another way of saying this is we're malleable. Here are two examples. The first is what occurs when you perform multiple sets of bicep curls over the course of a month. After about four weeks, you have the urge to wear sleeveless shirts...even in the arctic cold of a New England winter! Now why is that? The other example is when you break a bone in your leg and have to keep it in a cast over the course of the same month. At the end of this period, the leg on which the cast is wrapped has shriveled up to resemble a limp string of macaroni. In each case, the muscles have been *"remodeled"* to meet the demands placed upon them. And in each case the muscle selectively remodels its protein composition to permit energy to be used more efficiently when it contracts. So a muscle can be *"trained"* to work efficiently for longer periods if needed. Or, if not needed, the muscle recognizes this and shuts down protein production in the name of conservation. Whatever isn't required is then being conserved for the brain.

Booth and colleagues at Washington University in St. Louis, and elsewhere, discovered that mitochondrial content and capillary density in rats nearly doubled in skeletal muscle as a result of a four-month progressive running program. The researchers found that these changes in protein composition were enough to allow the otherwise sedentary animals to become *"marathoners."* How is this? The answer, it appears, can be found inside the cells.

You may have already heard of mitochondria. They reside within the cells of muscles and serve as the muscle's energy source, utilizing oxygen to make adenosine triphosphate (ATP) from the waste products of glucose and fatty acids. I'm sure you've heard of capillaries, too. They serve as pipelines delivering the much-needed oxygen to the mitochondria. When the mitochondria and capillaries double in numbers, this increase doubles the capacity of the muscle to make ATP with oxygen. This, in turn, provides an expanded aerobic capacity that allows the muscle to work for longer periods of time before reaching exhaustion. The increase in mitochondria also results in an increase in the size of the muscle. This is what happened to those biceps you worked out for four weeks and then just happened to showcase.

So we know that muscle can be molded to fit the demands placed upon it and this is done when the muscle recognizes a change in its usage. This change initiates an adjustment in the quantity of protein production in the muscle. To measure the expression of certain genes activated by exercise, Bengt Saltin and Henriette Pilegaard at the Copenhagen Muscle Research Centre and George Ordway at the University of Texas Southwestern Medical Center at Dallas collaborated with Darrell Neufer, an associate fellow in the John B. Pierce Laboratory and associate professor of cellular and molecular physiology at the Yale University School of Medicine, to conduct experiments on human research subjects using a modified Krogh one-legged cycle ergometer. The experiment was conducted in such a way that one leg of each subject completed 90-minute exercise sessions for five consecutive days, while the other leg resembled a couch potato, remaining still while its partner leg was cranking.

As you might expect if you've taken an introductory course in research methods, there was a control group and an experimental group. Muscle biopsy samples were extracted from the inactive leg (control group) before the exercise session on the fifth day and from the exercised leg (experimental group) prior to the fifth session, immediately after it and at various times in the 24-hour period when the sessions concluded. The two legs were then compared and the results revealed that a significant number of genes in the active leg's skeletal muscle were triggered from exercise.

The researchers identified three categories of gene activation and then concentrated their efforts by examining more closely the *"metabolic/mitochondrial enzyme"* genes. Although Neufer and his associates learned that these genes produce much lower concentrations of proteins, they also learned that the levels of these proteins remain for fairly significant periods of time afterwards —some even have half-lives for as long as a week. This metabolic/mitochondrial enzyme category of genes plays an instrumental role in muscle plasticity as reflected in the increase in mitochondrial and capillary concentrations that goes hand-in-hand with fitness.

As most of us know, exercise plays a role in weight management. When I ask clients what their training goals are at the beginning of a voluntary fitness program, many will express a desire to lose weight. This objective is becoming increasingly necessary as we continue to sink into more sedentary lifestyles. The percentage of overweight and obese people in the United States is increasing with each passing year, and we're now seeing children exhibiting the symptoms and effects of early-onset diabetes, a disease that was once called *"early onset **adult** diabetes"*.

As the U.S. trends toward weight gains, these gains move in lockstep with an increase in obesity and concomitant type-2 diabetes. This should come as no surprise, and it's not to the researchers who have studied this relationship of obesity to diabetes. Saltin et al hypothesize that the genetic adaptations for physical activity we've inherited from our very active hunting and gathering ancestors may very well be playing a role in both conditions.

The effects of exercise can be observed in something called the glucose transporter - 4 gene (GLUT4) that can be triggered by exercise without the involvement of insulin. GLUT4 allows glucose to cross the plasma membrane from blood into muscle cells. Why is this such a big deal? This crossing provides a way of providing energy to active muscle cells and, in the process, offers an alternative means for eliminating glucose from the blood. Without physical activity, the responsibility for getting rid of glucose falls exclusively on insulin and the pancreas that produces it. In due time, the sedentary muscle eventually becomes less sensitive to insulin, the pancreas is unable to produce enough insulin to compensate, and blood glucose levels spike, resulting in type-2 diabetes.

It's especially important to note that chronic diseases are a relatively recent phenomenon in developed countries. In the past century, there has been a significant movement away from infectious diseases (thanks to improvements in public health and discoveries in the medical and pharmaceutical fields) to diseases that are more chronic in nature, with the latter causing morbidity and mortality far more than infectious diseases did previously. Even with Covid, underlying metabolic comorbidities have been linked to most fatalities from the virus. We could do a whole lot better in a country that has the means to do so. But so far we're simply not paying attention. When we finally do, it's often too late.

Gabrielle Lyon, an osteopathic practitioner who has developed an approach to medicine that she has labeled *"Muscular Medicine"* and who was an undergraduate at Washington University where Booth has conducted his research, embellishes upon this concept of promoting the idea that our musculature serves as body armor. Muscles not only protect us from falls and allow us to push, pull, squat, lunge, rotate, balance, and hinge (we'll talk more about these in the third section of the book), muscles are critically important for processing the glucose buildup in our blood. As already mentioned, insulin eventually runs out if we don't allow our muscles to perform their necessary functions. We already know what the outcome of this is - it's type-2 diabetes, among other metabolic diseases. Our muscles actually protect us from these metabolic diseases.

Researchers studying this phenomenon wonder if the increase in chronic diseases is the exclusive result of our genetic makeup or might it be something else at play? The answer is *"it depends."* According to the Center for Disease Control, the answer is *"no"* if what we're talking about is disease-susceptibility genes - it's not like we're becoming more genetically exposed to heart disease, cancer or other chronic diseases. But the answer is *"yes"* if we are referring to genes whose expression is altered by our lifestyle choices. An example is the GLUT4 gene - for all intents and purposes, GLUT4 is a lifestyle gene. GLUT4 gene activation is directly affected by the degree of muscle contraction. Our inability (more accurately, our unwillingness until it becomes our inability) to be sufficiently active enough to have GLUT4 in the plasma membrane of skeletal muscle predisposes us to become pre-diabetic. This is on us.

We've already seen that weak skeletal musculature has been proven to pose a health threat to older individuals. A negative, downward cycle forms whereby an increase in the amount and rate of loss in size of skeletal muscle correlates very positively with the risk of premature death - meaning that the latter increases as well. John Morley of St. Louis University and others have written that a decrease in physical activity as we age appears to be the instrumental factor that results in weak muscles in our later years. A debilitating cycle forms between physical inactivity and muscle strength. Weaker and smaller muscles as we age (because we're doing very little in the way of movement) lead to a reduction in physical activity, with this reduction producing even smaller skeletal muscle, and on and on and on our way to sarcopenia - as well as increased susceptibility to metabolic disaster. As Dr. Ken Cooper reminds us, *"We don't stop exercising because we grow old – we grow old because we stop exercising."* We need more moving experiences in our lives in order for us to experience life in full form.

I'd like to make one final note about energy production before moving on. We've seen that our mitochondria serve as the power generators for our cells, producing energy that's transferred for use through our muscles…when we use them. It's important to emphasize that we don't produce energy on our own or out of nowhere…we get it from the sun through the foods we eat. The sun is our ultimate source of energy. So make sure the foods you consume spent sufficient time growing in the sun…and not in a laboratory.

CHAPTER 9

Moving Experiences

"Those who think they have no time for bodily exercise will sooner or later have to find time for illness."

Edward Stanley

MAYBE YOU'VE HEARD the story about the married couple who, thanks to practicing an incredibly healthy lifestyle, each lived well beyond 100 years before both dying of natural causes on the same day. They led such wholesome and righteous lives that the couple had a direct flight to heaven, bypassing purgatory and limbo and all the other checkpoints along the way. When they arrived on the first day, they were met with several surprises.

On the first morning, they go up to God and ask where the gym is. "Gym?" God replies, "You don't need to go to the gym here, you'll always be in perfect shape even if you never exercise." The wife says how nice that is, but the husband looks a little bit annoyed.

In the afternoon, they go back to God and ask where they can get high factor sunscreen. "This is heaven, you don't need it anymore, the sun can't burn you or give you cancer, enjoy the beaches." The wife is satisfied, but the husband starts looking genuinely angry.

Later in the evening, they go to God and ask where they can find a health food restaurant for dinner. "We don't have health food restaurants, you can eat as much as you want of whatever you want and never feel bloated or gain any weight."

Finally the husband snaps, and yells at his wife "You see?! You see?! If it wasn't for your bloody bran muffins, I could've been here forty years ago!"

How many of us would long for this heaven on earth... where we could pound IPAs and spiked seltzers all night and still possess the perfect body, roast in the sun all day for as long as we want without needing to spread gook all over us, and eat whatever and whenever and how much we want but never gain weight? How good would that be? Would you want it?

Well, I think some of us have been trying to replicate this kind of life on Planet Earth already and it isn't working the way God describes it happening inside the pearly gates of Heaven. It seems like we need to exercise if we want to be in *"perfect shape"*, wear sunscreen if we wish to protect our skin, and eat sensibly if we care to maintain a healthy weight. God is making us work for it here on the ground.

So move we must, like our ancestors frequently did. And this means exercise, a profane word in the English vocabulary for some of us. It's also a misunderstood word in that exercise isn't just what we do at the gym or on a cardio machine. Exercise comes in many forms, including simple physical movement, but many of these forms have become obsolete in the twenty-first century. We used to push mowers to cut our grass, shovel snow to remove it from our sidewalks and driveways, walk in the aisles to shop, prepare our meals from food we purchased or grew ourselves, wash and clean our dishes, and even wash and clean our cars. Much of what we once did required us to move about, to use our muscles. It required an expenditure of energy. Not now.

Kay Bowman, a biochemist and author of **Move Your DNA**, describes it this way - "*Motions that used to be incidental to living (occurring all day) and cellular loads that used to be built into everyday life have been doled out - to computers, machines, and other people on our behalf. There is no way to physically recover the specific bends and torques, no way to recreate one hundred weekly hours of cell squashing in seven, and no technology, at this time, smart enough to override nature.*" Amazon, UberEats...you name it... can deliver whatever we want right to our front doors. No movement is needed, except our thumbs to text the orders and our arms to bring in the prepared meals and deliveries from the front steps. With household chores, we fire up our snowblowers, jump on our lawn tractors, and turn on our leaf blowers if we haven't already farmed out these household chores to independent contractors - all in an effort to save time. Time for what? Tomas J. Philipson, an economist at the University of Chicago and a past member of the President's Council of

Economic Advisors, refers to it as the *"economics of obesity"* and I will address this more in a few moments.

Our work has become sedentary as well as we stare into computer screens all day or email our colleagues sitting just a few feet away from us. Just about half of all jobs performed in 1960 in the USA required at least moderate levels of physical exertion. Today that figure is less than twenty percent, and this translates into an average **reduction** of at least one hundred calories burned each day. This may not sound like much, but when multiplied by the number of days in a year (factoring in just work days), we're looking at over 25000 additional calories and about eight pounds of added weight...in just one year. This is why we need to hit the gym, or something that resembles it.

It's also why we need to find ways to keep moving frequently throughout the day. By now, we've seen this is a *necessary daily to-do item* if we have any desire to grow older in healthier ways. My mother used to refer to it as having *"ants in your pants"* for not sitting still. Exercise - and physical activity, in general - is actually a medicine that, when done correctly, has the kind of side effects that cause us to be... healthier, more vibrant, attentive, energetic, and optimistic in our outlook. The only costs are time and effort, albeit high costs for some. But what actually counts as exercise these days, is it the same as physical activity and how do we get to do either or both?

"Physical activity" and *"exercise"* are terms often used interchangeably but more accurately should be viewed as the latter being a subset of the former that contain similar

components while remaining somewhat distinct in character. Physical activity can be defined as any physical movement powered by skeletal muscles that results in energy expenditure measured in kilocalories.

In our day-to-day lives, physical activity can be grouped into job-related movement, various sports, fitness conditioning, household chores, yard work, and other related movement patterns (all of which, as already noted, we're doing much less of). Exercise, as somewhat distinct from physical activity, is defined by the National Library of Medicine as a subset of the latter that's *planned* (or should be) *in advance, structured, organized with an expressed purpose in mind that typically relates to the improvement or maintenance of one's physical fitness* (and we're doing even less of this). In the absence of general physical activity in our daily lives, exercise becomes even more essential.

I'm sure you know people who proudly boast to anyone who cares to listen that they *"don't do gyms"*, are allergic to sweat (their own and others'), and who sit on their recliners when they get the urge to exercise until such feelings pass. I hope you know by now, if you hadn't before picking up this book, that *daily* physical activity is required for life. You can blame this on our ancestors if you'd like (as we read in Chapter 8), but move we must if we wish to remain healthy human beings. Recall from the Foreword that, as we age, **the single most critical link to physical, emotional, and cognitive well-being is _physical activity_.** And this activity needs to occur frequently throughout the day if for no other reason than to rid glucose from our bloodstream. For those of us who claim we don't have time to do this, we should remind ourselves that we generally have a choice to make - *we either make time for wellness or surely we will need to make time for illness.* Haven't we already seen enough of the latter?

So the recommendation that we perform moderate exercise of some sort - typically it's walking that's recommended - for at least 150 minutes weekly (in thirty-minute increments five days a week) or 75 minutes of intense activity per week is actually misleading and underwhelming. I listen to people tell me they visit the gym just about every day, jump on the same elliptical machine or recumbent bike, and survive 30 minutes of moderately elevated breathing before returning home and either zooming all day in front of their computer screens or going to the office and doing something similar. In neither case is there much movement occurring for the rest of the day. (On a related note, I challenge the aforementioned approach in the gym as one that could be classified as exercise in the context of the definition of exercise - but more on this later.) In many respects, their bodies (and nervous systems) recognize this extended lack of movement as more like sedentary behavior and adapt accordingly.

We're actually sitting most of the day - in our cars, at our desks, in our recliners, on our couches. Sadly, we're often even sitting when we perform exercises on machines in the gym (more on this in the next section). But those who are completing their minimum required doses of weekly activity are faithfully following the recommendation of the health professionals. So why, they ask, are they not losing weight? Why aren't they getting more fit? It's because 150 minutes of movement isn't a sufficient replacement for *one hundred weekly hours of cell squashing,* as noted by Bowman.

Sitting for *most* of the day is really what our bodies experience. We negate the benefits of that thirty-minute dose of movement if we don't do much of *anything* else the rest of the day because our bodies typically adapt to what we most often demand of it. We're still, on average and as already noted, gaining one hundred additional calories per day. If you own a fitness device or subscribe to a service, this is why you receive those reminders to move *every* waking hour. As more *time-saving* devices and technology are introduced into our lives, the more necessary it becomes for us to *hunt for* ways to *spend* calories by using our muscles in frequent movement. Another feature on health apps and fitness devices is something called *activity minutes. We* should aim for a minimum of 100 active minutes each day over the course of time awake. That's less than ten percent of our time awake, and not even two hours, leaving eight hours for sleep (which may be generous).

A significant way we can increase our movement in the course of a day is to actually *be conscious of moving.* Here's why. James Levine, an expert on obesity at the Mayo Clinic, coined the term *"non-exercise activity thermogenesis"* (NEAT) to capture the energy we use to complete our normal daily activities. He found that we burn a decent amount of calories simply by existing. Our hearts, brains, and kidneys use up about 400 calories each while our livers expend 200 more. Then there's breathing, chewing our food, digesting our food...basic normal functions that require caloric energy. But Levine realized that we could burn so many more if we got up off our butts and moved around...an extra 107 just by standing and 180 calories by meandering about. One study had volunteers watch a normal evening of television but were instructed to get up and walk around during each commercial break. It resulted in an average of 65 calories burned in an hour and 240 in an evening. This can add up, right? (I know - that's four hours of television). Do it every night and we're dumping almost 1700 extra calories a week, and theoretically about a pound of weight lost every two weeks. Take note - it requires us to *be conscious of moving.*

NEAT can actually be a strong ally in our efforts to remain healthy. Various studies show that about fifteen percent of total energy expenditure in sedentary individuals comes from NEAT but can be as much as fifty percent in active people. Assuming that the typical person requires about 2500 calories daily, the increase from 15% to 50% results in a net difference of 875 calories expended. To put this in context with an exercise like running, the number 875 is twice what we'd burn if we jogged at a moderate pace for an hour. So, if you don't have time for the gym, well you can get your *moving experiences* in other ways.

There are more than a few other ways to ramp up NEAT in our lives. One way is to build more muscle. As mentioned in the previous chapter, muscle burns calories in a resting state because muscle is more metabolically expensive than body fat. Research has also informed us that possessing more muscle improves our body's ability to regulate blood glucose levels after we eat and this has been linked to reduced body fat levels. We've already observed this in previous pages.

Another way to increase NEAT is by increasing the intensity of our exercise routines. Higher intensity will require more oxygen which in turn will require more energy. The higher intensity will bring about excess *post-exercise oxygen consumption*, which simply means that our bodies continue to burn calories at a higher rate following an intense workout (more on HIIT in the next section). This translates into picking up your pace when walking, cycling, rowing...whatever it is. It's exercise that, literally, takes your breath away. It'll take more calories away as well.

Still two more ways are to increase your consumption of protein (anywhere from 20%-35% of the calories consumed from protein are used for digestion AND protein is needed for muscles) and to find more ways to move in the course of a day - take the stairs instead of the elevator, park at a longer distance from your destination, walk over to your colleague instead of sending an email, etc. In several of these instances, we're replacing time-saving decisions with calorie-spending activities. Do the cost-benefit analysis...the gains derived from NEAT may very well outweigh the relative cost in the time it takes to do it.

Not only should we be looking to complete at least 100 minutes of physical activity each waking day, you've also likely heard that we should be aiming to reach another number each day as well. It's 10,000 steps. This seems to be the standard benchmark for steps taken in the course of a day, and you'll likely reach 100 minutes of NEAT if you're covering at least 10,000 steps. But what's so magical about the number 10,000? How did we arrive at that figure?

The origin of this number actually dates back to 1965 when a Japanese company made a device it called *Manpo-kei*, which translates into *"10,000 steps meter."* The number 10,000 had less to do with any scientific reasoning and more to do with it being used as a marketing tool. The device took hold in Japan as people began using the number 10,000 as a step count to achieve on a daily basis. It wasn't long before researchers began studying the effects of that step count while assessing whether or not the number 10,000 was too high or too low.

There are claims out there that individuals can lose a pound of fat a week simply by covering 10,000 steps a day because of the potential to burn 3,500 calories from walking. This makes intuitive sense because a pound of fat consists of about 3,500 calories. If I can engineer an average caloric deficit of 500 calories over a seven-day period, then I've manufactured a deficit equal to 3,500 calories and, thus, a loss of one pound of weight per week.

Unfortunately, it's not so simple and this is simply because the amount of calories I may burn using the calculation of *10,000 steps a day equals 3,500 calories burned a week* is based upon my body type. Your body type may require more or less in the way of steps covered. Let's see how this works.

Body weight is the determining factor when calculating the number of calories expended when walking (or running). On average, heavier people require more caloric energy to move their bodies than do lighter people because it requires more effort to move a heavier object. If you've ever wondered how many miles 10,000 steps actually cover, estimates usually translate this figure into roughly five miles. So let's hypothetically say you weigh 180 pounds, then (based upon 200 calories burned per hour for a 180-pound human being) 200 calories multiplied by five miles equals 1000 calories. In a week's time, that adds up to 7000 calories and two whole pounds. This sounds promising. It's also really difficult to initially adjust to while maintaining your caloric consumption and juicing up your physical activity at the same time. But people do it, so...

Then again, it can also be done in more moderation and the intensity/distance can be increased incrementally each week. That said, this number of calories burned moves up or down in relation to your weight - you'll burn more if you weigh more than 180 pounds and fewer calories if you weigh less over the same distance covered. For example, if you're a string bean at 120 pounds, you're only burning 120 calories while your 180-pound walking partner is churning out eighty more.

Another important factor to consider is walking speed. As much as one's body weight determines calories burned in a designated period of time, so too does your pace. The faster we walk, the more calories we burn. It's that simple. And we've already seen the benefits of walking faster in previous chapters. Even if you're weighing in at 180 pounds, the calories you burn from walking depend upon your walking speed.

The Mayo Clinic sets the average walking speed at about three miles per hour. For a 180-pound individual, a leisurely 30-minute walk at two mph yields a caloric expenditure of 102 calories (as already noted), but crank up the intensity to a more aggressive pace of 3.5 mph for that same 30-minute walk and the caloric burn increases by 54% to 157 calories. *That's 110 more calories in one hour.* It can begin to add up over time. Why is that, you may ask? It's basic physics—it requires more energy to go at a faster pace, and this requires your heart rate to increase as it looks to produce the required oxygen to move your muscles. This means more calories burned covering the same distance. Look at it as a higher rate of return on your investment of time and effort walking (or running or doing any kind of movement). Think of Isaac Newton - a body in motion stays in motion. So get moving... because Newton also reminded us that a body at rest stays at rest.

But if shedding pounds is your primary objective when walking or performing any kind of exercise, it's critical to understand the nature of how weight loss occurs in order to adjust your approach accordingly. **We lose weight when we burn more calories than we consume - plain and simple.** If the amount of calories you consume in a day equals the number of calories burned, then the the net gain/loss is zero. The good news is you didn't gain weight. The not-so-good news is that you didn't lose any, either, if it's your intention to lose it.

To lose weight requires us to change the equation by creating an imbalance of calories consumed to calories expended. How do you do this? By increasing the duration of physical activity, turning up the intensity on your exercise, **and** reducing your daily calorie count. None of this is easy to do. Given our 21st century lifestyles, though, do we really have a choice *if* we care to be healthy and functionally fit as we age? It's a critical decision we all make - consciously or otherwise. Some of us may decide the price is too steep. It's a choice. Just know it's a choice because too many of us have thought for too long that it's not.

Here's a news flash, though... There actually may now be a third option available to us. Philipson, mentioned a few moments ago in reference to the *"economics of obesity"*, argues that we should have another choice available to us besides reducing calories and increasing physical activity. He is pushing drugs to get overweight and obese people to shed pounds, believing that the *"economics of obesity"* makes it virtually impossible for overweight individuals to trim down. He explains it this way in a piece he wrote recently in **The Wall Street Journal** - *"It isn't hard to see how obesity could become so widespread. There are strong incentives pushing Americans to gain weight. But this also means there is now a large global market for obesity treatments, which has inspired innovation."*

As already stated on previous pages, we're eating more processed foods that are produced inexpensively and we're moving less because our jobs have us tied to our chairs. It's a recipe for metabolic diseases and Philipson apparently doesn't trust that most people have it in them to introduce the antidotes - physical activity, exercise and a healthy diet - that will combat what he likely views as an insurmountable challenge for many of us to overcome. The World Health Organization estimates that about 650 million people world-wide were obese in 2016 and the World Obesity Federation predicts that almost a billion will be in 2025. Something needs to give.

Philipson sees the solution in giving prescription drugs to those in need, and there are a more of us in need each passing year. He points to two pharmaceutical companies that have recently marketed drugs for obesity and diabetes that regulate hormones to **reduce appetite**. The Food and Drug

Administration (FDA) approved Novo Nordisk's Wegovy in June 2021. The drug has been linked to an average of about a fifteen percent weight loss (a 250 pound individual will stand to lose 37 pounds). Eli Lilly's Tirzepatide was approved by the FDA last month to treat diabetes, but preliminary trial data show a weight loss of 22.5 percent after over 16 months (about 55 pounds in that 250 pound person). Those results, pointing to the research, were more impressive and statistically better at weight loss than observed with many behavioral interventions. The latter, behavioral interventions, are just as impactful but tend to lose their effectiveness once the intervention programs end and people return to the same *"economics of obesity"* behavior that initially placed them in these programs.

There's a problem, however. Wegovy went on the market with a monthly out-of-pocket price of $1,627. Medicare and several private insurers are hesitating to provide coverage because they see obesity as a **preventable disease** and, thus, the treatments are considered lifestyle drugs. Philipson feels differently and states that *"focusing on an increase in drug spending is shortsighted."* The American Diabetes Association estimates that the cost of treating diabetes in 2017 was $327 billion and two-thirds of this was covered by the government through Medicare, Medicaid and military medical benefits. Each one of these insurance programs impacts the national debt in significant ways. He goes on to argue that the additional costs of other obesity-related health problems like heart attacks, high blood pressure, strokes and some cancers are even more expensive and would be off set by the introduction of these, albeit very costly, weight-loss medications. Philipson views the cost-benefit analysis here as tipping the scale in favor of insurance coverage for these drugs. What do you think?

Here's what I think. I think there's another problem to consider. Weight loss without attendant muscle development raises at least one concern for me. Are we shedding pounds and simply becoming frail as we lighten our loads? Does this weight loss provide the same benefits that an increase in physical activity, muscle strength, and dietary changes would otherwise deliver to us? **Do we derive the same physical, emotional, and cognitive well-being without the physical activity? And is there emotional value in being able to manage our health and well-being through our own disciplined efforts?** I know that, personally, I derive a genuine sense of satisfaction when I complete my exercise regimen and walk out of my gym or any gym in which I may have worked out. It works for me. Obviously, I think it can work for you, too.

But you may be thinking differently now. You may be thinking you can actually experience that slice of heaven - eat as much and as often as you'd like, skip the workouts (but, sorry, you'll still need to wear sun screen) - with a daily dose of Wegovy or whatever. Maybe you see the cost easily worth the heavenly benefits derived from the pill, whether it comes directly out of your pocket or is a shared burden in the form of taxpayer support.

One final concern for now - remember back in Chapter 1 when I made reference to JFK and his advice - *"Don't ask what your country can do for you. Ask what you can do for your country."* Maybe this is worth repeating because we will soon be a nation with a lot of sixty-plus individuals residing in it. With over forty percent of our population heading towards obesity, will there be anything left in the federal piggy bank for much else? I think we need to get moving on this...and now.

There's an old Chinese proverb that goes something like this - *"A journey of a thousand miles begins with a single step."* It's also true that a journey of 10,000 steps begins with that first one...the one often most difficult to take. What's asked of us - to move daily and frequently - is not easy to do. But, like most things we find difficult to do initially, moving about actually does get easier the more often we do it. Even the 10,000th step can seem easier than the first because it's the latter that begins the journey outside of our comfort zones.

There's a lot of talk about basic individual freedoms these days. One that seems to have less and less interest for many of us is the ***freedom of movement.*** We willingly forfeit this freedom for the comfort of sitting on our sofas. We do this to ourselves, often unknowingly until trouble visits us. Let's face this - the joy of movement is lost to sedentary lifestyles. Could it be lost now to still another prescription drug? It remains an option and, thus, a choice.

I'm wondering this - does it necessarily need to be an either-or decision? Either I take the difficult road that can seem daunting or I take the pill? I wonder if the prescription could provide the initial boost for physical activity by helping us to reduce the weight we're lugging around and, as our loads lighten, we find it becomes easier to move about. We could be in a much improved position to move. Then, with the introduction of lifestyle changes and strength training in direct consultation with a health coach, a healthy change in metabolism could evolve and maybe we could incrementally wean ourselves off the prescription on our way to healthier living.

This is hard work and it, no doubt, challenges our comfort levels. What's necessary and what's not? The more often we make ourselves uncomfortable, the better we become at being comfortable with being uncomfortable. There is no doubt about this. But *why* would we make ourselves uncomfortable in the first place? And *how* uncomfortable am I willing to make myself? We'll talk about the importance of *"why"* and *"how"* up ahead in another chapter. For now, John Bingham, an American lawyer and politician in the early 1900s, helps with this advice - *"The miracle isn't that I finished, it's that I had the courage to start."* We'll develop this idea of getting started while getting used to discomfort more fully in the next section. And we will focus more directly on approaches to exercise as distinct from physical activity described here.

So it's looking like we may just have to admit eating those bran muffins are good for us, and that some discomfort in our lives - the hell we don't like - may actually bring us those heavenly moments of joy that make life so fulfilling. We may simply need to change our thinking about this, as difficult as we know changing our minds can often be, because muscles do matter. Or we can reject it all, say *"the hell with hell"*, and instead choose heaven in a prescription pill. Or a Big Mac. Who's right? Is there a wrong?

CHAPTER 10

Being Wrong Is Human

"Our love of being right is best understood as our fear of being wrong."

Kathryn Schulz

I'LL OPEN THIS last chapter of the first section with a throw-back to the Foreword and the quote that led off that segment - *"We don't see things as they are. We see them as we are."* I'd like for you to hold this quote open in a window on your mental screen while we delve into this next topic, one that will likely make you uncomfortable, although I may be wrong. Let's see.

If you've ever taken a developmental or child psychology course, you may recall the name Jean Piaget (a Swiss psychologist) and his early stages of cognitive development. Piaget's cognitive theory proposes that we construct mental representations of how the world works and how we interact with it. He labeled these mental models of the world *schemas*. Our schemas tend to become more numerous and detailed as we get older and we develop the ability to build complex mental models of our worlds. We have schemas to help us navigate our lives and to help us make predictions of what to expect. Without these mental representations, nothing would make sense. It would be akin to experiencing everything for the first time (which actually has several benefits - just not normally).

A central aspect of Piaget's theory is his emphasis on adaptation. Two processes typically occur when we take in information from our surrounding environments - assimilation and accommodation - and we use these processes by adapting the sensory information to our existing mental models. This is how we make sense of our worlds. We strive to match what we experience with what we *expect* to experience. We look to assimilate this new information into our pre-existing mental models. Makes sense, right? When it doesn't make sense, though, we get confused. We may even get pissed off. Things don't add up correctly. We're experiencing a WTF moment that's labeled *cognitive dissonance* in psycho-speak, the kind I experienced when I showed up for my first-year orientation at UConn. And we don't like how this feels. So what do we do?

In Piaget's developmental theory, the need for equilibrium is what fuels cognitive development. When we experience a new situation that can't be easily assimilated, disequilibrium occurs. We get knocked off balance. This brings on confusion, frustration, and a host of other negative emotions until we figure out what to do with this newly acquired information. We generally have two choices - assimilate the information into our pre-existing models, as noted in the previous paragraph, or adapt and create a new mental model that makes sense of it. We may need to *accommodate* the new information by creating new schemas. This takes a conscious effort...even willpower.

Once we adapt to new situations, growth and development usually follow. This is actually how we grow as human beings...when we adapt to new situations, we expand and develop new models. It's why I highly endorse novel experiences (that are legal and won't kill you). It's also not easy to do...which is why we often do everything possible to cling to our belief systems, even using *confirmation bias* to remain attached to what we *"know"* to be true so we don't freak out. This is also why we often tend to remain stuck in our known misery rather than confront our fears of what a leap of faith may bring.

Let's admit it - we don't like being wrong. In fact, Kathryn Schulz wonders in her exquisitely crafted book, **Being Wrong,** if *"we cling to our beliefs out of fear of being wrong rather than being sure we're so right."* Are we more concerned about revealing that we're wrong because we assume that people who are wrong are dumb, stupid, idiotic, clueless and possibly even evil? And we don't want to be perceived as such... even by ourselves?

Schulz reminds us that *"we're bad at recognizing when we don't know something, and we're very good at making stuff up."* She calls it *"confabulating"* - making shit up just to square our *"reality"* with our own personally-crafted mental models. We like to provide explanations even when the truth eludes us. We fill in the gaps with made-up stuff just to eliminate the angst that accompanies the confusion of wondering what the hell is happening. This is us applying confirmation bias to our perceived confusion.

Now is as good a time as ever to return to that window I asked you to keep open at the start of this chapter. I simply wish to remind you that *"We don't see things as they are. We see them as we are."* Our personally-crafted mental models determine how we feel and how we behave each and every day. Our mental models also inform us where we are, who we are, and what to do next. We see the world just as we expect to see it.

And we've seen by now what that world looks like that we "expect" to experience in our later years.

It's alright if we admit that we're wrong about this "expectation."

Schulz makes the point in her book that *"being wrong is a vital part of how we learn and change."* She goes on to emphasize that we're bad at saying *"I don't know"* but even worse at *knowing* that we don't know. Here's the thing, though - admitting that we don't know is the initial step in making change. It's also the first stage in cultivating wisdom. And it requires us to be comfortable with *not* knowing while we grapple with our novel perceptions and sensations until we finally do make sense of it all. Pema Chodron, an American Buddhist nun and author, counsels us with this advice: *"The truth you believe and cling to makes you unavailable to hear anything new."* Recall several pages back that I encouraged you to become comfortable with ambiguity. Well, here it is. Go for it.

Uncertainty is an uncomfortable position to hold for a very long time. But, as Voltaire reminds us, *absolute certainty is an absurd one to keep.* And William Faulkner advises us that we *"cannot swim for new horizons until you have courage to lose sight of the shore."* Ambiguity - not knowing - is an acceptable place to be...maybe even necessary at times...as a precursor to wise change and eventual growth. The challenge for us is to make our change a matter of identity rather than consequences when we eventually take that leap of faith.

A good deal of information has been presented thus far in this book that challenges our mental models of what it means to age in our current world. Some of this information may be new to you, and some of it you may have already known. Some of it may already be compatible with your mental representation of aging, some of it may be unsettling because now you're not sure what to think, and some of it you may simply reject as horse shit because it doesn't fit your existing mental model. Period. I still appreciate your interest here.

I mentioned in the first chapter that my hope is to provide a compelling argument that challenges our current notions of aging and what we're supposed to experience in our later years. I sincerely hope you're now at least open to the possibilities. I also hope you see that you may have been misled about how you're expected to live your life in your later years. *There are other options, other ways to experience how we age.* Perhaps you're willing to consider another form of reality.

We've reviewed research outcomes that help us understand why and how we age, and that there is no uniform standard on aging. Growing older, we've learned if we didn't know this already, is a pretty personal experience. We've also seen that our lifestyle choices can significantly help or hinder the way we experience the aging process, and that these choices can influence gene expression. We actually can regulate how our genes are expressed or suppressed. As for muscles, we need them because our lives - literally - depend upon them. But to change, as I cautioned you at the start, will take a concerted effort on a daily basis and it will mean getting comfortable with being uncomfortable. This is so much easier said than done. To start requires a rock solid trust in the process. A rock solid trust.

If you're not convinced of what's possible *yet*, I hope that you're at least no longer certain of what to expect. Seriously, I did remind you in Chapter 3 that we should be open to admitting we've been wrong about the aging process and that you'll need to be comfortable in that place of confusion. If you're thinking - *"I thought I knew, but now I'm not so sure"* - I'm totally fine with that. You should be, too. Stay here in this ocean of ambiguity while seeking *"new horizons"*. Keep in mind what the famous physicist Richard Feynman told us:

> *"I can live with doubt and uncertainty and not knowing. I think it is much more interesting to live not knowing than to have answers that might be wrong. If we will only allow that, as we progress, we remain unsure, we will leave opportunities for alternatives. We will not become enthusiastic for the fact, the knowledge, the absolute truth of the day, but remain always uncertain ... In order to make progress, one must leave the door to the unknown ajar."*

When you eventually come to the realization that change for the better is possible for you, the hard work that lies ahead may look daunting. You'll need to trust the process in order to take that leap of faith.

You may also be asking yourself, knowing what you now know, if the hell of discomfort is worth the heaven of contentment you get in return. *"Why"*, you may be wondering, *"should I put myself through this?"* Let's see if we can provide some support by mapping out how a new age of aging can become a reality for you. Let's see if we can find a new shore. Let's see if we can *accommodate* our way of thinking to seeing things as they really are…and not as we've been led to believe they're supposed to be. Let's see if we can find your *"why."*

PART TWO
INDIV-DUAL:
THE MIND & BODY AS ONE

CHAPTER 11

Starting Over: Find Your "Why"

"(S)he who has a why to live for can endure any how."

Friedrich Nietzsche

PERHAPS YOU'VE HEARD the story of a man who encountered three bricklayers one day working diligently with their hands. The man, curious about their behavior, asked the first bricklayer what he was doing. *"I'm laying bricks,"* the worker replied. He then went on to the second bricklayer and posed the same question. *"I'm putting up a wall,"* he answered. Finally, the inquisitive gentleman asked the third bricklayer and his response was, *"I'm building a cathedral."* Three bricklayers. Three perspectives. One with an authentic purpose. Can you guess which one?

A story like this is certainly open to interpretation, but the point of it is to differentiate busywork from work that's purposeful. If you were asked to choose the worker you think is most likely toiling away to collect a paycheck, then I'm guessing you'd select the first one asked. And if you were assigned the task of choosing the bricklayer who was committed to a deeper and higher purpose, I figure you wouldn't hesitate to select bricklayer number three. So tell me - what's the probability that the quality of work is the same among all three workers? Reminder - I said probability.

Much like the colleague you work with who sprints out the door when the bell rings to end the work day, I compare that first bricklayer to the gym member who begrudgingly treks to the fitness center and counts the minutes before s/he can bolt when the set time has expired. You know - the one who gravitates to the same elliptical machine, dials in 30 minutes, mindlessly plows through the measured time, and sprints out the door when the time expires, sometimes showing more energy on the exit than at any time during the exercise. The focus is more on time (let's get this done) and less on purpose (is there one?). The member pays little attention to what s/he is doing, likely has a vague objective - at best - of *"maintaining"*, sees little improvement and wonders why.

Conversely, the gym member who resembles the third bricklayer arrives at the fitness center with a specific plan that's part of a larger purpose. Time isn't the focus. The day's objective is. Each workout becomes a building block - a brick, if you will - with each one done purposefully, intentionally, and with full attention to the process. There are goals and objectives linked to a bigger *"why"* that provides the motivation to endure the discomfort that inevitably becomes an integral aspect of this experience. This gym member is building a cathedral, one workout at a time.

If you've ever frequented gyms, you've likely seen them both. Which one are you more of - the first or the third? As for the second bricklayer, I see that one resembling the client who initially seeks personal training because her doctor told her to lose weight (an other-directed goal) and whom you'll meet in a moment.

At the age of 72, and having presented Erik Erikson's stages of psychosocial development countless times in psychology courses I've taught, I find myself - somewhat surprisingly - at Erickson's final stage of *Integrity vs. Despair*. This is the period during which we reflect on our lives and the value we've derived from our life experiences (I actually spend more time looking forward than backwards but have found myself reflecting much more on my past since beginning this book project). *Despair* is the result of regrets while *Integrity* is reflective of a life well-lived.

For me, I have few regrets even though I've made a life's worth of mistakes along the way. I've made conscious efforts to learn from these mistakes, so they haven't been made in vain. This book is an attempt to share my experiences with a sincere hope that it helps you and others enjoy active lives until it's your time to check out. This is my *"why"* for writing the book. This is *"why"* I'm in a Starbucks on a Friday night in July struggling to find the words for my next sentence. It's a different *"why"* than the one that fuels my workouts. It's also much different in that I've had to start from the beginning with this, not sure of where it will go but trusting the process, nevertheless. It's never too late to start new...even at 72, although it's much better to begin earlier in your life than later when it comes to moving and exercising your muscles.

But starting over is really, really difficult and even harder when beginning something for the first time. Because we're not sure of where we're going or how long it might take to get there, doubt will likely seep in at the most challenging moments. Doubt will also leak in when we linger on the inevitable plateaus after what's often initial improvement, and we'll wonder if all this discomfort is worth it. Lingering on plateaus requires patience and trust, and is most certainly part of any learning curve.

So this brings us to the importance of finding **your** *"why"* with regard to exercise and physical activity. As Nietzsche tells us, *"(S)he who has a why to live for can endure any how."* If we know our *"why"*, the discomfort will become more tolerable...even more meaningful. I know my *"why."* Finding **your** *"why"* is the first challenge because goals need to have an emotional component for any chance of them to be realized. A rational, logical goal - like *"I want to lose weight"* - doesn't make the cut. **Why** do you want to lose weight?

We need to drill down with questions to get to the emotion that will drive the commitment. Below is an example:

Personal trainer: So, tell me, what are you hoping to achieve with your training sessions here in the fitness center?

Client: I want to lose twenty pounds.

Personal trainer: Great! I'm wondering *why* you want to lose twenty pounds?

Client: My doctor told me I needed to lose it. (an other-directed goal)

Personal trainer: OK. I'm wondering *why* he advised you to do this.

Client: Because he said I'm pre-diabetic and this could mushroom into something bigger.

Personal trainer: So this obviously concerns you and I can understand that you'd like to address this. Can you help me understand more specifically *why* you want to lose the weight? I know your doctor advised you to do this and you're following her recommendation, but I'm wondering *why* you're choosing to respond to this advice.

Client: I have two young children I want to see grow up and become adults. And I'd love to be a grandparent some day. (an inner-directed goal)

Personal trainer: That's awesome! You want to see yourself as a healthy human being going forward so you can be there for your kids and even for their kids, too.

Client: Yes. That's it!

Personal trainer: Perfect. Keep this vision of you as a healthy, fit human being as you embark on this journey. This will help you stay on the path when obstacles inevitably appear.

What we've done here is we've probed deeper with questions to identify the emotion (*the "why"*) that will drive the commitment. To change behavior requires an emotional commitment. Rational, logical reasons don't work, often times because they're other-directed goals. *I'm supposed to…is* ineffective, and so is *"I should…because"*. Substantive change has to get to the heart of the matter and, thus, must involve the heart in metaphorical terms. Emotions are heart-felt and not head-felt. After all, you call the love of your life sweet*heart* and not sweet head. Right?

Simon Sinik, a best-selling author, explains the importance of finding your why in his book aptly titled ***"Start With Why"*** by focusing upon what he refers to as *"The Golden Circle".*

It's comprised of three concentric circles, with each corresponding to a specific tenet of his theory.

The *inner circle* is your *"why"*, or your purpose…for getting out of bed in the morning, for going to the office, going to the gym, making lunches for the kids. Your inner circle represents your core values that should drive virtually every decision you make. Not coincidentally, it's attention to core strength in your exercise regimen that needs to occur first as well before moving elsewhere with your body. Core strength provides stability, both literally and metaphorically. The *middle circle* is your *"how"*, or the methods and techniques you will implement in order to fulfill your *why* - your purpose. For example, the *middle circle* includes the exercises and movement patterns you will perform on your journey (more on this in Part 3). Lastly, the *outer circle* comprises your output, or what you are achieving or wish to achieve. This involves the weight you're pushing and pulling, distances covered, time elapsed, etc.

As you can see with *"The Golden Circle"*, the *"why"* becomes central to the process. You behave with an authentic purpose when you connect your actions to the *"why"* that motivates you. In my role as a personal fitness coach, I can show you *"how"* to do the appropriate exercises for your desired goals, but they're meaningless without a genuine purpose - a *"why"* - for doing them. By connecting behavior to your *"why"*, you make your change a matter of identity rather than consequences.

Making change a matter of identity is rooted in human biology. Most all of us have an innate need to belong, to identify with something. We see this with political parties (Democrats vs. Republicans), coffee consumed (Dunkin vs. Starbucks), computers (Mac vs. PC), favorite sports teams (Yankees vs. Red Sox), phones we use (I phone vs. android), etc. We also see this with fitness memberships to niche clubs like Cross Fit or Soul Cycle or Pilates Plus or Yoga Centric or Peloton. The need to identify with something is an emotional pull that's rooted in our limbic brain. The appeal to belong is connected to this innate need and the choices we make are typically influenced by the *"whys"* we've created for ourselves that relate to the limbic brain. Sinik explains this in the context of how we make decisions.

Most decisions begin in our limbic brain, the part of the brain that relates to our feelings and that, in evolutionary terms, preceded development of our rational brain that we refer to as the neocortex. We may understand this better if we refer to the limbic brain when making emotional, *"gut"* decisions and the neocortex when making rational ones. (*A quick aside - the neocortex doesn't begin to develop until we reach adolescence, which may help to explain why teenagers do some of the craziest things and can't explain "why". And we see the limbic brain take control in adults after a few glasses of wine…who then do some of the craziest things and can't explain "why", either*) Anyway, the neocortex helps us with our *"have-to"* lists of things to do and our limbic brain is ready and willing to create those *"want-to"* adventures. The neocortex makes us rational beings. Really, which brain would you prefer?

Me, too. But there would be no guardrails to guide us through life without our rational brains. That said, a life devoid of emotion becomes a life-*less* experience. So we need to develop a compatible, working relationship between the two parts - our hearts and our heads - where we can both feel *and* think about decisions in our lives…a balanced perspective. It's also why we need to start the decision-making process in our limbic brains - the seat of our emotions.

Decisions made in our limbic brain are emotional ones - the *"why"* of doing anything. The neocortex then needs to make sense of the *"why"*, to operationalize it into a working *"how"* plan (sometimes the neocortex vetoes our *"want-to"* adventures). When we skip the initial step of identifying our *"why"*, we jump to the *"how"* phase that's controlled by the rational neocortex and make decisions based upon logic… like the client who initially disclosed that she was at the fitness center to lose weight because her doctor told her she should. This is an externally-driven goal. It's also logical and makes perfect sense. But it's incomplete. And the desired goal soon evaporates with the first setback. We're human **beings** more than we are *rational* beings.

Rationality is not enough to drive changes in behavior. The objective of being there for her changes when she links the behavior to the emotional *"why"* of wanting to see her children grow up to be adults and for her to experience being a grandparent. Originating from the limbic brain, the motive becomes inspirational rather than rational. In fact, the word inspire means *"to breathe into"* from its Latin origin. We breathe life into our rational goals, we inject inspiration and enthusiasm into what we choose to do. Our goals become internally driven. Everything changes when we break through to the emotional realm. We identify with our aspirations.

You've likely heard of SMART goals somewhere along your way through life. SMART is an acronym that guides us in making **S**pecific, **M**easurable, **A**chievable, **R**ealistic, and **T**ime-bound goals. This acronym has received a lot of play in recent years, both in schools with students and even in the business world. As Chip and Dan Heath remind us in their entertaining book titled, **Switch**, *"SMART goals presume the emotion; they don't generate it."* This is why we need to identify our *"why"* first before we devise any plan. SMART goals work when there's a *"why"* that propels them forward. Once we break through to feelings, everything changes and becomes clearer. And this new-found clarity can dissolve most kinds of resistance we'll inevitably encounter along the way.

So once you've identified your *"why"*, the *"how"* is the next step in this process. This next step involves logical planning that will support your efforts to realize your goals. Know this - you don't need to construct and orchestrate *every* step along the way. You just need to script the first few moves to get you jumpstarted. To attempt anything more at this point could be overwhelming. Like Horace told us - *He has half the deed done who has made a beginning.* Beginning is step one.

Let's do this. Find your *"why."* Why would you want to feel healthier, more energetic, more optimistic, more cognitively aware, more alert, and more socially connected? I don't know *why* anyone wouldn't want this - at any age and especially in later age development. But, that's me. You need to find your *why*.

Once you discover it and the authentic purpose your *"why"*represents, we can next examine habit formation and set you up for initial success by developing habits that escort you to your aspirations. This physical activity needs to be uncomfortable for you - there is no way around this - to derive the necessary benefits, and persistence through discomfort will require your *"why"* to be front and center. People will rise and grind in these circumstances as long as they perceive falling down as learning rather than failing on their way to eventual success. The right habits will go a long way in helping to build your cathedral.

CHAPTER 12

Our Habits, Our Selves

We first make our habits, and then our habits make us.

John Dryden

WE DON'T NEED to look long for examples of how habits provide structure and predictability in our lives and how changes to these habits - particularly those that are surprisingly abrupt and unplanned for - can trigger confusion, anxiety, and even depression. Just rewind to March 2020. That's when our lives were upended by an insidious enemy that wasn't even visible to the naked eye. Many of the habits we had in place to direct us through our daily doings suddenly worked no longer. We had to brace ourselves to adapt, not sure of what we were adapting to or knowing for how long we would need to shut down (remember we were initially told it would be two weeks?). This soon became a major-league-WTF moment for most all of us.

We could no longer kiss our loved ones goodbye nor even take a chance on hugging them. Forget about shaking someone's hand. Public transportation was a no-no as were Uber and Lyft. Plane rides? Nope. What did it matter, anyway? We really couldn't go anywhere. Very little was open. Gyms were closed and that was a major disruption for many people. Bars and restaurants were shuttered, too. That, as well, was a major blow. Arena lights were turned off and the games, concerts, and theater were halted immediately. That really sucked. We couldn't visit our doctors or go to school and work. We weren't allowed to…unless we were frontline employees. Parks were closed, play scapes roped off, basketball rims removed from backboards. Although we're taught that God is everywhere, we soon learned that we would be forbidden to visit with our Supreme Being in a house of worship. And forget about celebrating birthdays or other milestones in person with loved ones. What was left to do?

You know all too well. We zoomed and face-timed our way through the darkness. As for food shopping, that became an adventure for those who bravely ventured into grocery stores - masking up and keeping a safe distance from other potential lepers. Otherwise, we just ordered our groceries on-line and had our food delivered to us, but at our front doors so as to avoid human contact while keeping the virus at bay. We got crazy over toilet paper and cleaning materials and even produced our own hand sanitizer with grain alcohol. We got even crazier in our efforts to move up in line for the vaccine that would protect us from the viral enemy, calling in favors or fibbing about our age in order to cut to the front.

And then there were those who refused to get jabbed, guided by their own mental models for dictating their choice. With gyms closed, some turned to home workouts like Peloton and Peloton sold a lot more bikes and treadmills during the shutdown than they otherwise would have had life been *"normal"* as we knew it at the time. Those of us who chose to walk outside had to be cognizant of the *"enemy"* lurking on another's expelled breath, so we made sure that we crossed over to the other side of the road in order to keep our distance from what were once our fellow human beings. We were so vigilant. And so paranoid. These were uncertain times, with most of our routine behaviors no longer applicable in this dark, dystopian world.

Fast forward three years and it appears we've moved beyond the pandemic, even if we're not entirely sure that the pandemic is leaving us. Now that a *"new normal"* has emerged and we're still adjusting to a relative return to normalcy, I'm wondering how your life has changed as a result of this surreal experience we've endured. How have your routines been altered? You know - get up out of bed in the morning and then what? Commute to the office desk or to the desktop at home? Which means - get dressed to be seen in public or just from the neck up? Stuff like that. What new habits have you formed - good and bad? Are you eating any differently? What ones have you had to abandon that you've decided are no longer worth reviving? Can you explain to a casual listener why they're no longer worth it? And are there habits you're finally returning to after a forced hiatus? Finally, I'm wondering what impact this surreal time in shutdown mode has had on your mental models. Are you seeing things differently now? Has your sense of what's *really* important changed at all?

Recall that we addressed the influence of our mental models in Chapter 10 as they tend to direct how we *"experience"* our worlds, including how we interpret the information we receive from our surrounding environments. We see things as we are and not as they are. Why am I returning to this? Because you're in the process of forming new habits - your *how* - that will guide your behavior going forward, and this may likely mean you'll need to consider developing some brand new mental models - some new ways of seeing (including how you see yourself) - that correspond to your newly-formed habits in a way that you have had to adjust to the pandemic these past couple of years. Rather than assimilate, you'll need to accommodate by creating new ways of seeing. This means change, and we know that change is challenging to orchestrate. Why is this?

It goes back to what Piaget taught us - we seek equilibrium in our lives and our decisions are rooted in this balance. The habits we create, consciously or otherwise, support our quest for balance.

But substantive change is paradoxical because, by its very nature, change creates disequilibrium. In his classic book about the path to mastery that takes its title from the author's main focus - **Mastery** - martial arts expert George Leonard also writes about how we seek equilibrium, or homeostasis, in the way we go about our lives each day. We develop habits for how we do (or don't do) our morning routines, the way we commute to work, how we spend our lunch breaks, if/when we exercise and for how often, how we settle into our evenings and just about everything else in between. In due time, we construct our daily experiences in order to preserve our own versions of equilibrium. We form our habits so that they provide structure, routine, and predictability in our lives. *Once we form our habits, our habits then go on to form us.*

Here's proof - several studies conducted on habit formation report that about *forty-three percent* of a typical day for us is run on autopilot. We don't even need to think about what we're doing. It's automatic, so much so that Wendy Wood, author of **Good Habits, Bad Habits**, claims we wouldn't be able to list enough habits that would comprise *forty-three percent* of our day because we wouldn't be able to identify enough of them. We don't have to think because they are outside our conscious awareness. In so doing, we become more efficient just like our brains prefer us to be. Our mental models are serving our needs just fine.

So when we introduce change in our lives, we're intentionally disrupting our established equilibrium - for better or worse. If we lose our balance, our system naturally sets out to restore it ASAP. This is largely why change is so difficult. But we often make it more difficult by the way we introduce change. When we seek dramatic change in short order, our efforts backfire simply because our systems can't manage the magnitude of these disruptions to our normal routines and eventually force us back into our original patterns of habitual behavior. We find ourselves having bitten off more than we can chew. So we choke on our initial enthusiasm and feel like we don't have what it takes.

We do. We just need another way of doing this.

As juiced as we may be at the launch of a new initiative - in this case, developing an exercise routine and increasing NEAT - we can sabotage our efforts by being way too ambitious at the start. Recall that Michelangelo warned us about aiming too low and hitting our targets. Well, he was right on the one hand...and wrong on the other. It seems like we need to aim low with our first few steps in order to avoid the pull back to our *"normal"* patterns of behavior, or a regression to the *"norm."*

Think about it - how many have you known, perhaps you included, who have embarked on an ambitious plan - any plan - and have seen it derailed because of a major setback early on? For example, you commit to running two miles three days a week and doing strength training on three other days. That you haven't run two miles since before the pandemic arrived and have never really lifted weights ever before is irrelevant. You're pumped to achieve your goals and are determined to jump right into it. What often happens?

You get injured, of course, because it was too much to take on too soon. Your internal system that regulates equilibrium couldn't manage the increased load and, in response, shuts you down. Leonard explains it this way, *"Resistance is proportionate to the size and speed of the change, not to whether the change is a favorable or unfavorable one."* It's a case of too much too soon and not good vs. bad. Or it may simply be that you soon lack the motivation to continue after (say) three days, so you quit. We need to adjust our mental models in order to make change favorable to our systems because as Jim Ryun, the accomplished distance runner and former Congressman, tells us, *"Motivation is what gets you started. Habit is what keeps you going."* The habit needs to make sense. We simply can't rush the process. Instead of plunging right in head first, it's better to tip-toe in feet first.

It turns out that there is an optimal pace of growth that evolves naturally for most all of us when managed properly. Virtually all systems, human beings included, detest radical change that occurs abruptly. I mean, we experienced this first-hand in March 2020. Burn the candle at both ends, as my mother used to say, and soon enough those two ends will meet. Push the body too hard and too soon - lifting too much weight, running too far/too long - and it will revolt even sooner on us. Cramming doesn't work. We just need to find our own optimal rate of growth. How?

By taking it slowly at the beginning. I know - it sounds counterintuitive. But sustainable progress requires allegiance to an optimal pace of growth. Peter Senge, the business systems guru and author, puts it this way: *"Virtually all natural systems, from ecosystems to animals to organizations, have intrinsically optimal rates of growth. The optimal rate is far less than the fastest possible growth."* You can't help but want to get there as fast as possible when you launch a new initiative, but you need to understand that going slowly will actually get you there faster because you'll avoid the injuries that impede progress along the way. We all have our own personal rate and this may require some trial-and-error approaches to probe our limits. As for writing this book, there is a natural and optimal pace to follow. I write every day so as to reinforce the habit of writing, with some days being more productive than others. Especially early on in the process of cultivating new habits, consistency is far more important than intensity. Keep in mind the **act of doing...**and do it consistently.

When I'm experimenting with new routines for myself, the initial phase of any new venture - and this includes anything novel that I attempt in my own gym - is intentionally performed slowly. Any increase I introduce in my exercise routine is no more than ten percent (weight, distance, time) of what I have already been doing. Additionally, any new lift that I execute - added weight or a different movement pattern - is performed slowly so that I can 1) remain in control of the movement, 2) allow my nervous system sufficient time to *"figure out"* the execution of it, and 3) pull out of the movement if I need to before it's too late and I injure myself. As for injuries, these occur when our nervous systems don't recognize danger in time; thus, the slow tempo when introducing new stuff. By the way, I employ this same approach when working with clients.

James Clear develops the idea of growth rate optimization in his best-selling book, **Atomic Habits.** He calls for a focus on small daily wins and *one-percent* improvements that nudge us along the way to our desired goals and aspirations. A perfect example of this nudging can occur in the gym when strength training - lift weight that's too light and your muscles go unchallenged while lifting too much will result in an injury. It requires you to find the optimal weight that will appropriately challenge your muscles to stimulate growth (remember mitochondria?) while keeping your system in relative equilibrium.

I actually implemented this approach over two decades ago when I imploded personally, likely the result of me dealing with my father's death. It was a case of overtraining with my internal monitoring system shutting me down because I wasn't listening to my body. Chronic fatigue set in and I was both an emotional and physical wreck. After giving myself eight weeks to rest and recover, I returned to the gym and began using 2.5 pound dumbbells to bench press. This weight was, literally, one percent of the 225 pounds I had been pressing before I tanked. Slowly, I worked my way back, incrementally increasing the weight each week. Approaching it this way allowed me to avoid injury and return to the gym the next day...and the next day...and the next (For the record, I do not bench press 225 pounds today because my tendons and ligaments won't tolerate it. So I've lightened the load considerably and increase the number of repetitions instead).

This is very similar to a technique used in cognitive behavior therapy that's labeled *covert desensitization* wherein the therapist guides the client incrementally towards a feared behavior or object so as not to overwhelm the individual's equilibrium - like, for example, flying on airplanes. Several steps are planned out that gradually nudge the client ever so slowly to the airport, through security, and on to the plane. This typically takes several sessions to realize. When I work with clients, it's precisely the same approach I use. I'm probing the boundaries of one's comfort zones, venturing just outside those limits in order for the system to adjust accordingly without revolting and instead allowing for incremental progress. We're nudging growth along the way. In due time, this growth becomes significant. I repeat...in due time.

When done properly, it works. We can return to the gym the next day instead of making an appointment to see a doctor. Fitness training should be designed to simultaneously improve our functional fitness level while reducing our probability of injury - in the gym and in our NEAT movements throughout the day. The right habits, as Ryun reminds us, will keep us going. After all, it's often injuries that derail our efforts. We can easily fall victim to the mindset that *"if some is good, more is better."* It's not. In this case, especially early on, some is good. Period.

I realize we've been talking about habits without actually defining them in operational terms, so let's do this before moving on with designing those that stick and help make us healthier human beings. According to a 2012 study published in the British Journal of General Practice, habits are *"actions that are triggered automatically in response to contextual cues that have been associated with their performance."* We're well aware of the automatic nature of habits - that we perform them without really thinking - but I especially want you to keep in mind the importance of *contextual cues* related to habitual behavior because we'll be elaborating upon this more in the next chapter.

We've already addressed why new habits are so challenging to establish (preserving equilibrium), yet we haven't mentioned why some habits may be more difficult to hack than others nor have we differentiated good habits from bad habits...although the latter may be a subjective interpretation in that productive habits can morph into counterproductive ones when we take them too far (I'm thinking of the Greek motto - *"Nothing in excess, everything in proportion"*.) But what's too far? That's up for debate and for each of us to decide.

It shouldn't surprise any of us that bad habits are typically pleasure-based habits. They deliver heaping doses of dopamine, that much desired chemical neurotransmitter in our brains that creates pleasurable sensations and upbeat feelings, and these sensations are what prime our pumps to repeat the specific behavior for even more of this chemical high. It's the reinforcing reward that we experience when eating fast food (processed food is engineered to provide instant gratification, with the McDonald's french fries melting in our mouthes upon immediate contact being a primary example), smoking (instant nicotine rush) , consuming drugs and alcohol, gambling (even *"almost"* winning gives us a buzz) and when on social media. Just the mere scent of cinnamon wafting through the mall from the Cinnabon counter, intentionally distant from the food court so that the smell will be distinctly picked up by our senses, stimulates production of dopamine.

It's the Pavlovian effect - ring the bell, deliver the food pellet. Do it enough times and we begin salivating at the sweet odor wafting from the Cinnabon counter. Refined sugar does this to us very effectively and is added to a whole host of foods today in order for us to experience the sought-after sugar high. *"Comfort food"* gets it done for us just as successfully. In each case, the sense of immediate gratification is experienced. The instant buzz we derive from these pleasurable experiences relate directly to the pain-pleasure relationship that we'll address in a few chapters. Here's a hint though - a bad habit may be when we experience the pleasure up front and then feel like shit afterwards. Can you think of any examples? I bet you can. Yet we continue to repeat these behaviors for reasons we'll soon discover.

The reality is that we form bad habits in the same way that we form good habits. *"The general machinery by which we build both kinds of habits are the same, whether it's a habit for overeating or a habit for getting to work without really thinking about the details,"* says Dr. Russell Poldrack, a neurobiologist at the University of Texas at Austin. Both types of habits are based on the same kind of brain mechanisms. Go for a smoke or go for a run. Doesn't matter. It's the same sequence...stimulus - response - reward.

It's just that the immediate gratification that dopamine provides with our *bad-and-I-know-it-but-it-feels-so-good* habits is what makes it much more difficult to crack them. A few puffs or a couple of sugar cookies and I'm where I wish to be. To get to a similar place by jogging requires me to move my ass. It's that imagined feeling of discomfort that gets in the way. It's also the effort involved. Quick buzz vs. *"I have to push my body and feel like crap for 30 minutes to get a similar high?"* Is this really a choice? Poldrack explains it this way - *"If you do something over and over, and dopamine is there when you're doing it, that strengthens the habit even more. When you're not doing those things, dopamine creates the craving to do it again,"* Poldrack says. *"This explains why some people crave drugs, even if the drug no longer makes them feel particularly good once they take it."* Even, as mentioned in the previous paragraph, if it makes us feel like shit afterwards we still want it.

I know - it's not easy to get rid of a bad habit. There is a way around this, however. Victor Frankl hinted at this with the following observation - *"Between stimulus and response there is a place. In that space is our power to choose our response. In our response lies our growth and our freedom."*

Although we may be creatures of habit, we also happen to be more than nonthinking, mindless critters. We actually have a complex brain structure, as we've already seen with the neocortex and limbic brain, that possesses the capability of exerting willpower and self-control in our day-to-day decision making. We have it within us to override that wished-for immediate hit of dopamine. After all, people do it, right? *"Humans are much better than any other animal at changing and orienting our behavior toward long-term goals, or long-term benefits,"* reports Dr. Roy Baumeister, a psychologist at Florida State University. Baumeister views self-control in the same way he sees muscles - *"Self-control is like a muscle. Once you've exerted some self-control, like a muscle it gets tired."* And this can drain us of the willpower we have in our possession which, by the way, is a finite amount. Of course, much like a muscle, the more we exert self-control the better we also become at being more disciplined human beings. Like the Nike ads tell us, *"just do it".* The more often we **do**, the more self-control we're able to exert and the more the habit becomes ingrained. Remember what I wrote just moments ago - consistency is more important than intensity early on in the process. But, clearly, this is much easier said than done or else we'd all be *just doing it* already.

So getting back to this complex brain in our possession, sometimes the different parts of it compete with each other, as we've already observed with the limbic brain and neocortex. The hard truth is that some of the brain's mechanisms are more amenable to change than are others. When we act *"instinctively"*, what we're really doing is being instructed by our *non-conscious* mind (as distinguished from the unconscious mind). On the other hand, we exercise *conscious* executive-control functions when faced with decisions that require willpower. The latter involve cognitive processes that evaluate and monitor our actions.

For example, starting a new job requires conscious attention to policies and procedures until they become *"second nature"* to us. These tend to be thoughtful, planned, clearly articulated efforts to execute a deliberate action. This takes conscious thought and a degree of willpower, with the latter determined by the degree of difficulty the action poses. New habits need to begin here in the conscious realm. The exercise of willpower can initially be - literally - exhausting. Remember - willpower is *not* inexhaustible. We need to use it wisely. It's really why we need to employ the *one-percent rule* in our progress. It's also why we need to re-arrange our environments for success to occur.

So let's delve more deeply into habit formation, with our conscious minds and executive functioning in the forefront. How can we form enduring habits that are linked to our *"why"* and that produce more satisfying experiences for us in place of those that deliver pleasure in the immediate moments? How can we cultivate confidence in our ability to stay on our chosen course of action and pick ourselves back up when we've experienced the inevitable setbacks along the way? How can we change to become the person we envision and to put into practice our *"why"* for taking on this challenge? There is a way.

CHAPTER 13

Empowering Habits

"Consciously create habits because habits
unconsciously dictate your life."

Anonymous

IT'S AN ANNUAL ritual for many of us. Come late December, we resolve to change our lives for the better with a New Year's resolution and, if we're feeling really ambitious, we'll throw in another one or two for good measure. Usually these feel-good intentions relate to some form of self-improvement, whether it's losing weight, exercising more, reducing stress, getting more organized, saving money, or eating better. Whatever, we commit to making these changes with the advent of a new year because it's a convenient marker for a fresh start. We resolve to be better human beings. Next year **will** be the year we do this. Really. Beginning *"tomorrow"*.

And then what happens along our way to July?

In spite of our noble intentions, research coming out of the University of Scranton a few years back suggests that only about *eight percent* of us actually achieve our New Year's goals. Another study published in 2016 revealed that *forty-one percent* of Americans still make these annual resolutions anyway, and yet another study appearing back in 2007 indicated that *fifty-two percent* of these seemingly well-intentioned human beings expressed confidence that they actually **would** achieve them (meaning, obviously, that *forty-eight percent* weren't sure…not a promising sign).

So let's look at the typical success rate in the first six months of a new year. Exactly *three-fourths* of these ambitious individuals are holding steady after one week, *seventy-one percent* remain committed after two weeks, and this southbound percentage over time continues as *sixty-four percent* still have a grip on it after one month while just *forty-six percent* are rockin' steady after six months. In the end and after twelve months of trying to get better, we're back to the aforementioned *eight percent*. This may not be all that surprising, but, still, do you ever wonder why we're so bad at this?

Of course, there is research to help us understand why we are. In one 2014 study examining reasons for failure, *thirty-five percent* of participants who punted on their New Year's resolutions reported that they had, in hindsight, set **unrealistic goals**. You have to appreciate their candor. *Thirty-three percent* of those who failed indicated that they didn't maintain a record of their progress (so how do you know then?). This next data point may be the most logical and compelling reason of them all - *twenty-three percent* admitted they **forgot** their resolutions. Seriously. Lastly, about *ten percent* of respondents disclosed that they had made too many resolutions and it simply became impossible for them to track.

So, let's review reasons for failure... setting unrealistic goals, inattentiveness to progress (no journal, etc.), and establishing too many goals. This all makes perfect sense when keeping in mind what we considered in the previous chapter with habit formation. Too much too soon...and not paying attention. If you're thinking I neglected to mention the *twenty-three percent* who forgot their goals, I didn't. I just can't imagine they were all that serious in the first place.

We seem to know that it's not just poor planning and inattention that doom our efforts. The real reason, we believe, is that we lack sufficient willpower to get the job done. We're simply too weak in the face of temptation. This is what we think. So we beat ourselves up for being wimps. But how would you feel if research tells us that we're wrong when we do this to ourselves? It's not self-discipline that we're lacking, it's actually something much simpler. What?

"OK," you're thinking, *"I have my **why** for putting up with this exercise bullshit that's going to make me hurt initially but eventually make me feel better, and I know that I need to take it slowly at the start. Oh, and I have a plan too. That should do it"*...or so we think...until the muscle soreness might be something we don't recognize and we become concerned and so we better back off before we get really injured and...before we know it, we're right back to square one. I know this - I've seen it with my own clients and with friends/acquaintances. As Michael Goldblum, playing a journalist in the 1983 movie *"The Big Chill",* put it so wisely, *"We can go a day without sex, but we can never go a day without rationalizing."* It's a talent we all seem to possess and one that comes installed at birth for most all of us. This is the point when we call ourselves

wimps and then we lapse into becoming what we think when it's really are already-existing (mostly bad) habits that tend to pull us off course.

Remember that habits exist outside of our conscious minds and work in ways that are much different from when we're hanging out in our conscious realms. Wood (**Good Habits, Bad Habits**) describes this as the *"second self"* because it operates independent of the self we know. Recall that we would be challenged to list all of our daily habits that comprise *forty-three percent* of our day simply because we're not even aware we have them. We just *do* them. But think about it - shouldn't we pay at least *occasional* attention to what we're doing almost half the time? How does this happen, anyway? *"If this is the case"*, you may be wondering, *"can I get to do my daily dose of exercise without actually thinking about it?"* Believe it or not, you can...once you establish an exercise habit.

Rather than retreating internally and doubling down on our willpower when our self-control wanes in the face of new challenges, we instead need to look outward at our environments and the *"friction"* they're creating as obstacles. What's friction? It could be our old habits, for example, that we can so easily default to...when the contextual cues are right in front of us (like our beds at the end of the work day, but just for a *"quick"* nap...or a couple of cookies that won't hurt because, after all, the plate is just a short reach away). Or it could be other people (kids, spouses, work colleagues) who grab our time just when we're about to exercise. Changing environments can change habits, and they can reduce the friction along the way. Kurt Lewin, the German-born American social psychologist and a pioneer in social and organizational psychology, explains it this way - *"Contexts are our environments and they generate forces upon our behavior."* Self-control gets really simple when we realize that it involves putting ourselves in the right situations…the right environments… to develop the right habits. In so doing, habits take the place of self-control. They're done automatically…without thinking.

Eventually, you can exercise without really having to think about it. How long will this take? The research says that an enduring exercise habit takes, on average, 91 days to form. That's one day at a time…repeated ninety-one times. On the 92nd day you don't have to think about it…you just do it.

So for a solid exercise habit to form after 91 days, it requires (assuming your **why** is in place*)* the right contextual cues, immediate rewards, and a consistent effort. *"It's mainly by establishing and maintaining stable patterns of behavior rather than by performing single acts of self-denial that self-control may be most effective,"* states Roy Baumeister, another social psychologist that we first heard from back in Chapter 12. Implicit in stable patterns of behavior is the act of consistency. Remember - consistency is more important than intensity early on. We need to practice doing it, whatever *"it"* is.

I mentioned several pages back that I used to rise and grind in the dark so I could be at the gym no later than 5 am and arrived more often at 4:30 am because I lucked out with the gym opening earlier. Why then? Because there was very little friction getting in the way (except for the warmth and comfort of my bedsheets, particularly in the winter). The rest of the world was sleeping, including my children and work colleagues, so nothing would be getting in my way. I performed my habit at the same time each day. And the *"reward"* was the intrinsic sense of achievement I felt for having completed my objectives. I also experienced a rush of positive emotions upon exiting the gym, likely the result of of an endocannabinoid high that we once attributed to endorphins (more on this coming up). I had the energy I wanted and was ready for my day as the sun rose in the East. The most difficult part? Getting out of bed...and then one step at a time to the car and gym. Context - workout clothes laid out on floor, work clothes hanging in the car, coffee prepared, repetition - same time each day. It's the contextual cues appearing in that space between stimulus and response (remember Frankl?) that are critical. These need to be placed strategically.

Early on, executive-function thinking needs to take hold. Remember the quote that opened this chapter - **"Consciously create habits because habits unconsciously dictate your life."** You may need to override already-existing habits that may cause friction and replace them with contextual cues that trigger your desired behaviors. This requires conscious thought. What will you be doing? When will you be doing it? How will you reward yourself? So the first few steps need to be scripted, but they don't have to be perfect.

Charles Duhigg, author of **The Power of Habits**, maintains that successful habit changes begin with experimentation that reveals the cues and rewards that drive your habits. He suggests a four-step process that relies upon identifying your routine(s) and experimenting with various rewards in order to effectively isolate your cues and understand why you embrace these habits. **Step One** - record your habit-driven routine, detailing each step from beginning to end (Judson Brewer - a neuroscientist

- takes this a step further in his book, **The Craving Mind,** suggesting we employ mindfulness or meditation to help us develop conscious awareness of the specific routines that encapsulate our habits); **Step Two** - switch out rewards to discover your cravings. In other words, change the reward each time you're about to engage in your habit and record the first three words you think of when you're doing this to capture how you're feeling at that moment; **Step Three** - use categories to identify your cue. This will assist you in determining the trigger for this habit you're trying to change. Duhigg claims that all cues fit into one of five categories...location, time, emotional state, other people, and what's occurring at the moment you're about to engage in the habit. It's not uncommon for an underlying emotional issue to be driving the impulse; **Step Four -** head off temptation by changing up your cues. Clear, in **Atomic Habits,** elaborates by encouraging us to not only remove cues that are getting in the way but we should replace them with more positive cues to spur behavioral change. The visual cues should be visible and directly related to your burgeoning habit.

Begin where you are and **resolve to move yourself out of your comfort zone.** If you're already performing an exercise routine, review it and determine what needs to change (Part Three of this book may help you with this). If you're a *"walker",* resolve to pick up your pace and extend your stride. An anaerobic pace is one that - literally - takes your breath away. Aim for a minimum of ten minutes of this pace at least three times weekly. Look to gradually extend this *"out-of-breath"* experience by ten percent each week (adhering to the optimal rate of change). You, too, should refer to Part Three for suggestions on how to incorporate strength training into your routine.

Schedule your workouts in your day where there is the least amount of friction. Keep a journal…it holds you accountable (I have journals I've kept that go all the way back to the 1980s). If you happen to miss a planned session, record it. Lastly, choose a plan that's realistic and doable. Set yourself up for success and review it after six weeks. You need to feel confident that you can achieve your goal and you need to believe that your efforts will get you there. Trust the process. Keep your *"why"* in front of you.

Let's not forget NEAT movement throughout the day. You can begin to pair a bathroom break with a long walk around the office before arriving to call on nature. Or you may take the stairs to the next floor instead of the elevator. I recently lived in a seven-story condo building and would walk the four flights necessary to reach our place. I didn't have much success, though, trying to get residents to incrementally increase the floors they could climb. For too many, one floor was too much (not really, but it's what they believed). Get a treadmill desk if you find it impossible to leave your work station. Hunt for opportunities to move. Stanford researcher BJ Fogg, author of **Tiny Habits: The Small Changes that Change Everything,** began doing two pushups each time he went to the bathroom. That led to lots of other small habits, like having eggs and spinach for breakfast, and he ended up losing 20 pounds in six months.

Aim to incorporate regular movement throughout the day until you don't have to think about it anymore. Begin with where you park your car. For example, I park at the end of the lot no matter where I am…going to the gym, the grocery store, the movie theater. Look to build brief 10-15 minute bouts of walking during the day. Most of us are in sedentary positions, so you'll probably need to *"hunt"* for your opportunities to move. I know...I've had to do this. Another suggestion is to build movement cues into your environment. This could be, for example, a BOSU in the corner of your office or resistance bands hanging on your bedroom door. Make it an objective to move in the morning before you even get out of bed by lightly stretching and then taking a short walk around the house. Mow the lawn with a push mower. Walk the course - even with a pushcart - when you're playing golf. And, speaking of golf, learn to counter-train against habits you repeatedly perform...in the case of golf, perform exercise rotations that are the opposite of a golf swing. We will address this in greater detail in Part Three, but know that you should incorporate pushing, pulling, squatting, lunging, hinging, rotating, and balance into your daily routines in order to optimize your functional fitness.

Yes, I know, taking care of ourselves is a full-time commitment. But the converse - not taking care of yourself - can eventually become a full-time obligation as well when you spend your days attending multiple doctors' appointments and otherwise dealing with the discomfort that a sedentary life is most certain to deliver. I'd rather spend the time taking care of myself. Wouldn't you rather as well?

CHAPTER 14

The Value of Voluntary Pain

*You must go through that short-term pain to reach
long-term gains. A meaningful life is about growth,
not comfort.*

Maxime Lagacé

A FRIEND OF mine is often quick to point out that nobody he observes running is ever looking like they're enjoying themselves in the least. *"Why would anyone do this? They look like they're in absolute agony"*, he'll regularly remind me. Faces grimacing, sweat dripping, lungs panting, legs aching from burning muscles. *"If they really enjoy what they're doing,"* he muses, *"shouldn't their faces reflect it? Shouldn't they be smiling while they're running?"* What's my reply? *"Are you smiling when you're having an orgasm?"* Wait, what? Think about it. It's the subject of this chapter…not orgasms, but the value of voluntary pain that accompanies a meaningful life. It's an important topic to consider…the pain-pleasure relationship… at this point in your journey. Why? Because you are inviting voluntary pain into your life when you embark upon a challenging exercise regimen…if done correctly. I'll explain the orgasm reference, by the way, up ahead.

So have you ever wondered why we take on challenges that can be frightening, exhausting, bring on sadness, and that can even hurt like hell? There are several ways we do this to ourselves on a fairly regular basis - getting on amusement rides like roller coasters, watching horror movies that scare the bejesus out of us, even sad ones that create steady streams of tears. I like hot peppers…really hot ones. My family really doesn't understand why, especially when I accidentally rub an eye after handling one. It just doesn't make any sense to them when I say that the buzz I get after the burning subsides is a potent high that makes the brief pain well worth it.

And then there are those of us who take on extremely physical challenges like running marathons or even ultra-marathons, grinding through triathlons, lifting weights, hiking treacherous trails, climbing steep mountains, or participating in heavy-duty boot camps. No smiles here. Why do we choose to inflict so much pain upon ourselves? Wouldn't life be a lot more enjoyable on a couch in front of the television with a bag of chips and favorite beverage in our grasp?

Well, most of us would probably agree that life could certainly be more pleasurable on that couch, but in no way would it be more meaningful. In this life we live that's filled with so many uncertainties and existential angst, we need to seek challenges like the aforementioned in order to invite meaning into our lives. I mean, think about it - which provides more satisfaction (not to be confused with pleasure) for you…those chips and drinks you just polished off (feel free to replace it with the treats of your choice) or the three-mile run you just slogged through? I bet you may not even want the treat after you've run. You're buzzing already. You'll see why in a moment.

There are other ways we introduce meaning into our worlds that also involves struggle. Some of us decide to have children. Those of us who make this decision and are fortunate enough to bring this experience into our lives are certainly not seeking pleasure. It's no block party raising kids. That said, it can be incredibly satisfying and rewarding to sacrifice ourselves for the good of our children and to see them grow into healthy, fully-functioning adults. We also choose to take on demanding career roles that can be highly stressful on our way to professional success and status (this can be potentially problematic when our core identity is wrapped up in our career role). Or we may decide to devote our efforts to caring for an older parent, even taking her/him into our homes for them to live. We may volunteer with organizations like Habitat for Humanity. There are lots of ways we can add meaning to our lives. The philosophers tell us that a life well-lived is one filled with meaning. So what's this mean?

Accepting that meaning naturally involves the pursuit of significant and impactful goals, suffering will most assuredly accompany meaning (a central tenet of most religions, by the way). Refer to the examples I just provided in the previous paragraphs to recognize that conflict, anxiety and perhaps even more distressing emotions come hand-in-hand with meaningful pursuits. As Paul Bloom reminds us in his engaging book, **The Sweet Spot,** *"when one chooses to have a child or go to war or climb a mountain, one might not wish for or* *welcome suffering…but it always comes along for the ride."* We don't ask for suffering, but we should come to expect it in our pursuit of meaningful engagements. It's the feeling we experience when we exit the gym after a solid, purposeful workout. Indeed it's this suffering that instills in us a sense of pride, achievement, and well-being when we actively engage in such pursuits, pursuits that I will remind you are fueled by our *"why"*. It's also what you miss if you decide to access your slice of heaven with either of the two weight-loss drugs you should recall from back in Chapter 9 - Wegovy and Tirzepatide. I have already alluded to this.

Here is a little known secret - there is a strong link between pleasure and pain that is deeply rooted in our biology. At a fundamental level, all pain causes the central nervous system to release endorphins, proteins that actually serve to block pain and otherwise mimic opioids like morphine to stimulate feelings of euphoria.

Let's return to the runners that my friend is so quick to ridicule for a pertinent example. Bouts of high-intensity exertion naturally release lactic acid, a by-product of the breakdown of glucose when we're in an oxygen-deprivation mode (exercising while short of breath is classified as anaerobic conditioning - you're sucking wind). These runners feel the burn when they've pushed themselves beyond their comfort zone in such a way that their muscles are unusually challenged; thus, the face grimacing, lungs burning, etc. The lactic acid stimulates pain receptors in their muscles, and these communicate their *"suffering"* to the brain through electrical messages sent via the spinal cord. The signals are interpreted as a burning sensation in the legs, usually causing the runners to downshift on their pace or even shut down altogether.

And then the nervous system's control center, the hippocampus, kicks in. This portion of the brain responds to pain signals by triggering the production of the body's own pharmaceutical agents called endorphins. The proteins of the endorphins bind to opioid receptors in the brain and head off the release of chemicals involved in the transmission of pain signals. This, in effect, assists in blocking pain. But endorphins do even more by activating the brain's limbic region – the same area activated by just about anything passionate. It's an **after**-pain rush that resembles the high of morphine, which also binds to the brain's opioid receptors.

Concurrently, the pain of high-intensity exercise also triggers an increase in still another of the body's arsenal of painkillers that's referred to as anandamide. Known as the *"bliss chemical"*, anandamide binds to cannabinoid receptors in the brain (more on our endocannabinoid system in an upcoming chapter) to squash pain signals and bring on the pleasurable high that resembles cannabis. Cannabis, you should know, binds to the same receptors as does anandamide. This is what's referred to as the *"runner's high."* Previously thought to be only an endorphin buzz, more recently this high has also been attributed to endocannaboids and we'll elaborate upon this in an upcoming chapter.

But before we go any further, we need to distinguish between pain we experience that is uninvited and pain that we voluntarily take on. It's the latter that is the subject of this chapter and a term has been coined by University of Pennsylvania psychologist Paul Rozin and Kendra Pierre-Louis at Aeon to describe this willing acceptance of discomfort that they call *"benign masochism."* They define it in this way - *"Benign masochism refers to enjoying initially negative experiences that the body (brain) falsely interprets as threatening. This realization that the body has been fooled, and that there is no real danger, leads to pleasure derived from 'mind over body.'"* In other words, we derive pleasure from seeking out pain with our endeavors while simultaneously recognizing that it won't cause any serious harm. We connect the pain to that which delivers us pleasure and eventually we bypass the pain and link the activity exclusively to pleasure. This is what the runners are doing when they accelerate their pace.

Rozin and Pierre-Louis, by the way, inform us that the ability to experience benign masochism is a uniquely human trait. Animals aren't capable of doing this. Try bringing your dog, for example, on a roller coaster ride...you can be sure that Lassie won't have any interest in getting on it a second time. *"Generally, when an animal experiences something negative, it avoids it,"* explains Rozin.

Let me remind you of that conversation I had with my friend where I ask if he's smiling when he's having an orgasm. This isn't as far-fetched as you may be thinking. The link between sex and pain has been revealed in a study conducted by Barry Komisaruk from Rutgers University whereby researchers used fMRI to picture the brains of women as they stimulated themselves to climax. What they discovered may blow you away in that they found more than *30 areas of the brain were active, including those involved in pain*. Another study discovered that cancer survivors who had nerves severed in their spinal cord to relieve chronic abdominal pain lost the ability to have orgasms. If their pain returned, so did the orgasms. Komisaruk believes that there is a fundamental link between pain and orgasmic pathways. *"Another observation is that the facial expressions during orgasm are often indistinguishable from those in pain,"* he says. He has photos of each that are indistinguishable to back up his claim. When I share this with my friend, he doesn't know how to respond. Do you?

Another research outcome provides clearcut evidence of the intimate relationship that pain has with pleasure. A study of acetaminophen determined that the over-the-counter drug certainly does its job of relieving pain, but it also dulls feelings of pleasure. In this particular study, students were given either acetaminophen or a placebo and were asked to evaluate the intensity of their emotions towards a series of provocative pictures. The research results revealed that the drug blunted the highs as well as the intended target of the lows – strongly suggesting that pain and pleasure operate on shared biological pathways.

For us human beings, then, it certainly seems like the pain we look to eliminate in our lives has the unintended consequence of lessening the pleasure we experience as well. It's a deal we strike with ourselves, isn't it? In our effort to reduce pain, we proceed to reduce the effects of **all our emotions.** By doing so, we become comfortably numb. Recall the effects of NSAIDs (over-the-counter pain medications) and their long-term use eventually creating a counter effect of increasing our pain over time. The message is - if you're looking to reduce pain in your life, know that you will be reducing pleasure at the same time. It's a trade-off that requires a cost-benefit analysis we all must consider when managing our emotional lives.

Let me remind you that it's not just over-the-counter painkillers that produce this kind of blunting effect. Several prescribed medications, as already noted in Chapter 5, do the same. When we blunt our senses, we diminish our ability to take in information about our surrounding environments through these same senses. We suppress our engagement with life and we lose our proprioception. This is what helps to make us *"old"* too soon. Those who are taking multiple medications (remember poly pharmacy?) are particularly vulnerable. It doesn't have to be this way. There is another lane.

I briefly referred to a book written by Paul Bloom, **The Sweet Spo**t, a moment ago and wish to elaborate more upon what Bloom writes about with regard to the pain-pleasure relationship. Wonderfully entertaining and conveyed in a conversational tone, Bloom lays out three basic premises - 1) certain types of suffering can be sources of pleasure, 2) a life well lived is more than a life of pleasure…it involves, among other things, moral goodness and meaningful pursuits, and 3) some forms of suffering, involving struggle and difficulty, are essential parts of achieving these higher pursuits. A central theme of his book is that at least some degree of misery and suffering is absolutely essential to a full and meaningful life.

Bloom makes reference to Michael Inzlicht and a term the latter coined *"the effort paradox"* wherein we'll often choose to do something over doing nothing, and the effort itself can become a source of pleasure. The way the world works, according to *"the effort paradox"*, is that rewarding experiences often require work and this effort, which may begin as a negative experience, gets paired with the reward and then becomes rewarding in itself. The takeaway is that *if you suffer for something that gives you joy, soon the suffering itself can provide you the joy you seek.* This is what the runners are experiencing. And this is what happens with our newly formed habits.

So we can view pain in a more favorable light in that negative and positive experiences (pain and pleasure) are not opposites. How is this possible? The answer rests in the human capacity to interpret and respond to experiences/events in the surrounding environment.

Remember Shakespeare? *"There is nothing either good or bad but thinking makes it so."* Or Milton - *"The mind is its own place, and in itself/Can make a Heav'n of Hell, a Hell of Heav'n."* Even the Tao Te Ching weighs in - *"Happiness rests in misery/Misery hides in happiness/Who knows where they end."* It becomes a matter of interpretation that can change over time. To persist, pain has to have meaning. Eventually we link the activity that initially causes us pain to the eventual pleasure we derive from it. I exercise for the endorphin and anandamide high and not the discomfort I experience while getting there. I'm not thinking so much about how I feel as I enter the gym (that said, I do a quick assessment as noted in Chapter 3) as much as I'm looking forward to how I'll feel when I exit it and for the rest of the day.

Bloom titled his book **"The Sweet Spot."** Here's why. Our choice to suffer is not for naught. Suffering, no doubt, has its risks, both practical and moral. But, still, Bloom argues that chosen suffering experienced in the right way, at the right time and in the right doses adds value to life. **It's the right amount of suffering that matters - not too much and not too little; thus, the sweet spot.** For me, the Greek ideal comes to mind - *Nothing in excess, everything in proportion*. Recall the rate of optimal growth? Chosen suffering can bring us profound pleasure and, as we've seen here, is an essential part of the experiences we deem to be meaningful. At its fundamental core, suffering is part of the human condition. Know your *"why"* for your suffering. This is what give meaning to it.

Finally, it should be noted that the order in which we perceive events matters with regard to how we recall them. To quote Daniel Kahneman, an author and noted psychologist - *"When we look back on an event, we give extra weight to how the experience concluded."* In other words, we're more inclined to assess an experience by how we recall it and we're typically influenced in our recall by what we *last* experienced. With pain and then pleasure, we recall the pleasure.

In the end, know this - those of us who pursue both meaning **and** pleasure are the happiest among us. Go ahead and have that cold beer **after** you exercise…you'll link both as a pleasurable feeling that follows the discomfort of the workout.

The proper dose of pain + pleasure + meaning = Happiness. It's there for your taking. Go get it with physical exercise and move your body through discomfort to arrive at that slice of heaven we're all seeking in some way or another. Exercise is medicine, the most effective antidote you'll find for a whole host of issues. You've surely heard the phrase *"No pain, No gain."* The **right** amount of pain will deliver the **right** amount of gain…it's the optimal rate of growth that is in play here. You may be grimacing on the outside, but you're smiling on the inside. Find your sweet, sweat spot - that balance of pain with pleasure - and stay in it.

CHAPTER 15

The Obstacle Is the Way

Falling down is part of life. Getting up is living.

SHIT HAPPENS. NOBODY escapes it. Nobody. Accidents occur, people screw up, people screw us over, we get fired, get seriously sick, we injure ourselves or others injure us - physically and emotionally. We may accidentally step in a hole and twist a knee, or reach up to grab a dish from the top cabinet and tweak our back. We could go to bed feeling perfectly fine and wake up feeling like death warmed over. Illness can arrive unexpectedly. Or we get a medical diagnosis that totally shocks us. We may even hurt ourselves as we push too far beyond our comfort zones with a new exercise regimen. Whatever. Just know we all get knocked down at various points in our lives no matter what. But believe it or not, this actually may be life's intention, as you'll see shortly.

Even the most prepared human beings on the planet suffer from unplanned events that we call setbacks. When they do, it may feel like living just plain sucks and there seems to be no way out. There is, of course, and it's the subject of this chapter. It's about our **responses** to the obstacles we inevitably encounter. We may not control the latter, but we most certainly have total influence over the former. Shit will happen while you challenge yourself and establish healthier habits. Expect it. At some point. Just know that **how you respond** to the expected setbacks will make all the difference for you going forward.

So let's take a closer look at what happens when we encounter an obstacle. If you're like most people, including me, you probably experience a whole host of emotions, with none of them bringing you any joy. Initially, you may get depressed. You may also get angry. *"Why me? Why now?"* Frustration can set in. Even worse, you may give up hope, thinking that what you're facing appears insurmountable, or it wasn't meant to be, or you simply don't have the energy to fight through it when what you were attempting to do - a new exercise routine, for example, designed to create the best version of you - was already difficult enough. I know that each time I get seriously injured, my immediate thought is - *"Is this it? Is this the one that knocks me down for good?"* That's my first thought. But if I stay stuck in depression, anger, and hopelessness, you tell me - how will this type of thinking, this mindset, help me to move forward? Or you? It won't.

Here's another aphorism you can post somewhere in times like these - ***Grow through what you go through***.

After my first thought revealed in the previous paragraph, my second is - *"Get a grip here. Let's find out what I'm dealing with and figure out how to fix it."* The setback that's viewed as an obstacle becomes the way forward through this challenge.

The obstacle, in effect, provides the springboard for action…
if you embrace it and don't run from it with painkillers or use
"comfort food" to soothe your pain or alcohol or whatever.
We've already seen how frequent use of painkillers can blunt
all emotional feelings and can also exacerbate our pain rather
than relieve it. Remember - it's your *"why"* that fuels your efforts. You need that *"why"* more than ever during times like
these.

Perhaps you recognize this passage from a classic movie
spoken by a people's hero a couple of decades ago - *"Let
me tell you something you already know. The world ain't all
sunshine and rainbows. It's a very mean and nasty place and
I don't care how tough you are, it will beat you to your knees
and keep you there permanently if you let it. You, me, or nobody is gonna hit as hard as life. But it ain't about how hard
ya hit. It's about how hard you can get hit and keep moving
forward. How much can you take and still keep moving forward. That's how winning is done."* Look familiar? (If not, the
answer is at the end of this chapter.)

Moving forward…that's what it's all about. But moving
ahead and cultivating growth isn't linear. In other words, a
graph of our improvement over time would likely be a mix of
jagged and straight lines rather than a slanted one on, say, a
45-degree angle. The jagged lines represent the fits and starts
we experience along the way…two steps forward, one step
backward. The straight line depicts the plateaus we're typically on while building for next-level gains. This is generally
how learning and growth occur. But just like we gain strength
in between our workouts and not during them (we create
micro-tears in our muscles during exercise and our built-in

mechanisms repair these tears while laying down more muscle fiber in between workouts), the same is true when we encounter these inevitable setbacks. We mistakenly confuse growth with success when, in reality, it's our failure that fuels our successful efforts (success and failure operate along a continuum much like, as seen in the last chapter, pleasure and pain do). The setbacks and failed experiences force us to consider alternatives, to expand our vision, to think in new ways that could lead to better solutions. This ultimately leads to growth. It's staying comfortable in that place of ambiguity - have you heard this before? - while you figure out your way forward. Growth doesn't occur if we remain mired in depression, anger, and hopelessness. We need to take action…and the right kind.

I'll provide a couple of examples of the many in my own life as they relate to this concept of failure/setbacks forcing us to examine situations from other perspectives. These examples are all fitness related because this is a book that is emphasizing the several benefits of physical activity. I've already shared with you my response to a debilitating back injury I suffered seven years ago - developing a strong core to protect my lumbar spine. I also mentioned in the first few pages here that I had drop foot (a feeling that resembles your foot being *"asleep"*) for seven months caused by a pinched perineal nerve in my lower leg. I was in my early fifties at the time. This setback led me to water - pool workouts have turned out to be awesome strength, cardio, and recovery workouts for me that I only discovered because of the drop foot. With this injury, I also came to the realization that muscles are nothing without nerve stimulation to activate them. In each instance, I chose to focus upon what I **could do** rather than dwell on what I couldn't...once I moved past my initial frustration, sadness, and anger. I'm not looking for any trophies here for doing what I've done. I'm simply sharing examples. I'm sure you can provide your own examples as well.

And then there is simply the benefit of slowing down, of reassessing our lives, from a setback caused by illness or injury because you've likely heard the phrase that *"illness and injury are the Western forms of meditation."* For many of us, it's the only time we ever apply the brakes on our otherwise hectic pace and give pause to contemplate what our lives are actually like. We can even get seriously ill and begin to question, however brief this may be, our own mortality and the time we have remaining in this life. Serious setbacks have a way of forcing us to reassess our priorities in life. The main takeaway is that there are lessons wrapped in obstacles and our focus should be on actionable objectives rather than wallowing in self-pity. There is a way out. We simply need to be open to possibilities and pay attention to them.

You may recall the name "Marcus Aurelius" from your high school World History class. If you forgot, know that he was a powerful ruler when the Ancient Roman Empire ruled over the world. He was also, at times, philosophical and contemplative and he offered his own perspective on setbacks - *"Our actions may be impeded but there can be no impeding our intentions or dispositions. Because we can accommodate and adapt. The mind adapts and converts to its own purposes the obstacle to our acting. The impediment to action advances action. What stands in the way becomes the way."* Aurelius was echoing the tenets of Stoicism, with the Stoics known for flipping obstacles upside down. Rather than retreat from the

171

obstacle, Marcus encourages us to embrace it and grow forward with it. Easier said than done, but it is necessary for us in order to grow in our lives.

The obstacle is the way is actually the title of a very popular book written by Ryan Holiday in which he provides several examples of well-known people throughout history who have acted upon Aurelius' advice. Appropriately titled *"The Obstacle Is the Way"*, Holiday weaves the tenets of Stoicism through his stories and highlights its three basic principles - 1) **Perception** - the first response to a setback needs to be one of awareness, one in which we take the necessary time to perceive the situation *objectively* (removing emotion from our perception) and to accurately describe the obstacle in front of us; 2) **Discipline of Action** - this involves taking constructive action to move us beyond the obstacle, and herein lies the lesson in that the action we take would likely not have been anything we would have considered doing until we were faced with the roadblock (consider the examples I provided); and 3) **Discipline of the Will** - through this experience of perceiving the obstacle and then taking action, the Stoics remind us that we are building internal strength and fortitude...willpower, if you will...as we work our way forward.

When we subscribe to this philosophy, everything that happens to us offers an opportunity to improve our position in life. In effect, the shit that occurs provides us the compost for our continued growth. Recycle the compost and use it to grow yourself. Even Ben Franklin advised us that *"the things that hurt, instruct."* Franklin sounds like he could be speaking about what we addressed in the previous chapter, doesn't he?

So, we've established that shit happens and nobody avoids it in life. We don't have control over the shit that happens, but we most certainly have complete control over our responses to it. We may need to recall the words of E. E. Cummings, first shared here in the Foreword, during times like these - *""It takes courage to grow up and become who you really are."* The setbacks - obstacles - that occur in our lives provide opportunities for us to behave in different ways, to do things differently. So expect them. And be ready to respond courageously with objective perception, the discipline of action, and the discipline of your will. Falling down is part of life. Getting up is living.

I'll conclude this chapter with an old Chinese proverb titled *"Good luck? Bad luck? Who knows?"* that may help with putting misfortune and setbacks in proper perspective.

Many years ago a wise farmer lived in China. He had a son who was the apple of his eye. He also was the proud owner of a fine white stallion horse that everyone admired. One day the barn in which his horse resided caught fire and the horse escaped from the barn and disappeared. The villagers came to the farmer one by one and said: "You are such an unlucky man. It is such bad luck that your horse escaped." The farmer responded: " Who knows. Maybe it's bad, maybe it's good." The next day the stallion returned followed by 12 wild horses. The neighbors visited him again and congratulated him on his luck. Again, he just said: "Who knows. Maybe it's good, maybe it's bad."

As it happened, the next day his son was attempting to train one of the wild horses when he fell down and broke his leg. Once more everyone came with their condolences: "It's terrible." Again, he replied: "Who knows. Maybe it's good, maybe it's bad." A few days passed and his poor son was limping around the village with his broken leg when the emperor's army entered the village announcing that a war was starting and they were enrolling all the young men of the village. However, they left the farmer's son since he had a broken leg. Everyone was extremely jealous of the farmer. They talked about his sheer good luck, while the old man just muttered: "Who knows. Maybe it's good, maybe it's bad."

Good luck? Bad luck? Who knows. Time will eventually reveal this to us. In the meantime, just get up, lift your head, stand tall, and keep moving forward.

(Answer to the question posed on page 207 - Sylvester Stallone, Rocky)

CHAPTER 16

The Endocannabinoid System: How It Works

"There were never so many able, active minds at work on the problems of disease as now, and all their discoveries are tending toward the simple truth that you can't improve on nature."

Thomas Edison (1902)

HARDLY KNOWN TO the vast majority of people, including many medical professionals, is a system that resides within us that regulates a multitude of functions and looks to maintain internal homeostasis throughout our bodies. It's labeled the endocannabinoid system (ECS) and the name is derived from the plant that led to its discovery - namely, cannabis. The ECS is formally known as the endogenous cannabinoid system (endogenous is defined as within the body, meaning that we produce our own cannabinoids - seriously) and it plays a critical role in our overall health and well-being, with its complex actions conducted in our nervous and immune systems as well as in all of our body's organs. The ECS is, quite literally, a bridge between our bodies and minds, and it's included in this section for that very reason. Each of us, I remind you, is an indiv/dual…consisting of both mind and body that are inseparable.

As you might expect, the connotation imbedded in the name has invited misleading and pejorative references since it was first discovered in 1992. But it has been slowly gaining credibility in recent years with more research being conducted on the ECS as cannabis continues to be legalized for medical and/or recreational use in an increasing number of states. Legalization has reduced the stigma surrounding both substances and has made it much easier for researchers to access both CBD and cannabis. Still, much more remains to be discovered about the ECS and the effects of both CBD and cannabis on the ECS.

So let's take a closer look at where the ECS is located in each of us and how it functions to protect us. The ECS itself is comprised of three component parts - endocannabinoids, receptors in our nervous system and around our bodies to which endocannabinoids and cannabinoids bond, and enzymes that assist in breaking down both endocannabinoids and cannabinoids. Endocannabinoids are the substances our bodies naturally produce in order to stimulate the aforementioned receptors, with the two currently best understood being anandamide and 2-arachidonoglycerol (2-AG). We've already touched upon anandamide - *the bliss chemical* - in Chapter 14. Cannabinoids, on the other hand, are what we introduce to our ECS by external means through cannabis and/or CBD consumption.

As mentioned in the first paragraph of this chapter, the ECS functions to preserve homeostasis - balance, harmony - throughout our internal environments while all sorts of distractions are occurring outside of ourselves. The ECS kicks into action when it recognizes that something internally is out of whack and it works to restore harmony. How?

Let's return to our runner in Chapter 14 who is panting, grimacing, and straining to push forward...all while beginning to sweat profusely. The ECS recognizes that s/he is overheating and immediately takes action to cool the runner down. The ECS conducts this via cannabinoid receptors found in specific tissues; thus, the sweating. We have two types of cannabinoid receptors (and possibly more as researchers continue to learn about the ECS): **CB1** that are located in our central nervous system (brain and nerves of the spinal cord) and **CB2** that are found in our peripheral nervous system (nerves in our extremities), the digestive system, and specialized cells in our immune system.

Cannabinoid receptors are believed to be among the most plentiful in our central nervous system, and the ECS assists in regulating a whole host of functions through these receptors, including our appetite, immune function, sleep, memory, mood, motor control, digestion, temperature regulation (as already observed with our runner), inflammation, and - last but certainly not least - pain and pleasure. That's a whole lot, isn't it?

Our bodies activate the ECS in precise ways such that it does exactly what is necessary and nothing more. Once the endocannabinoids complete their tasks and return our bodies to a homeostatic state, specific enzymes then arrive to decompose these endocannabinoids in order to make certain they do no more than is needed. The system and process are both efficient and effective in doing their jobs of establishing balance internally.

Phytocannabinoids are plant substances that stimulate cannabinoid receptors, and THC is one that's likely familiar to many in that it's the active component in cannabis. But another phytocannabinoid that's received a ton of attention in recent years from both researchers and the populace at-large is cannabidiol - or CBD. As you may know, CBD doesn't have any psychoactive properties (which is why it's sold legally provided that the level of THC in the CBD is below .03 percent, even in states where cannabis is not legal), so its many potential benefits are experienced without the psychoactive high of THC. One specific function of CBD in the brain is to stop the FAAH enzyme from deconstructing anandamide, so the latter can provide a more powerful impact. It's precisely why CBD has become a viable option for treating anxiety disorders, among other ailments - including inflammation. You may recall that I mentioned in the Foreword my occasional use of CBD.

Given its relative importance in regulating our internal environments, it's worth mentioning here that a deficiency in endocannabinoids may cause a whole host of problems. This has been labeled clinical endocannabinoid deficiency (CECD). Know that CECD isn't a disease in and of itself but is rather an umbrella term that includes conditions with this common feature. Three conditions have been identified with CECD and you've likely heard of each one - fibromyalgia, migraine headaches, and irritable bowel syndrome. These conditions have been labeled *"functional conditions"* or *"central sensitivity syndromes."* As you may know if you have suffered from any of these conditions, they have been resistant to several treatments. Thus, researchers are evaluating the efficacy of cannabis-based interventions for these painful ailments.

Cannabinoids are being researched as potential treatments for all kinds of conditions, not just those involving endocannabinoid deficiency. Some of the illnesses being researched include Alzheimer's disease, cardiovascular disease, acute and chronic kidney disease, chronic pain conditions, chronic inflammatory diseases, autoimmune diseases, as well as neurological, neurodegenerative, and psychiatric illnesses. CBD is also currently in use for pediatric epilepsy, pain, inflammation, acne, and asthma. So it's apparent that the ECS, in concert with appropriate dosing of CBD, may offer potential benefits for a wide range of conditions.

I wish to reiterate the importance of appropriate dosing here. Much like we've already emphasized the value of finding our sweet spots with regard to exercise (not too little and not too much, but just the right amount to stimulate growth) as well as the appropriate amount of voluntary pain that will deliver subsequent pleasure, the same holds true with CBD dosing. Remember always that whereas some may be beneficial, consuming more may be harmful to your health and well-being. This is due largely to the receptors in our brains that receive and process the external cannabinoids. Incrementally increasing the dosage can eventually lead to a concomitant increase in tolerance, developing the need to increase your dosage in order to experience the desired effects previously felt. When this occurs, you've moved past your sweet spot and have entered harmful territory. You've simply gone too far because you've then made your own endocannabinoids useless - not a healthy consequence. Take notice…and adjust accordingly. If/when this occurs, consultation with a physician who is qualified to certify individuals for medical CBD use as well as with pharmacists working at dispensaries is absolutely necessary. Not recommended. Necessary.

At this point in time, it's unlikely that your own doctor(s) understand(s) the potential benefits derived from cannaboid/CBD consumption simply because it's never been addressed in medical schools. I've asked several doctors, specialists as well as generalists, about their knowledge and awareness of the ECS and I've not yet found one who knows anything about it. It's neither included in the medical school curriculum nor in pharmacy programs (one pharmacist I spoke with indicated that it was offered as an elective choice). Given this, they're understandably not in a position to advise in the proper indications, dosage, and route of administration. They are behaving responsibly in this regard, as much as the preference would be for them to be more knowledgeable. Having said this, know that, among the various sources I've used to research ECS and attendant cannabinoid use, two prominent sources have been the Mayo Clinic and Harvard Medical Review. I'd say they're reputable sources. Wouldn't you?

In spite of the two largest U.S. physician associations - the American Medical Association and American College of Physicians - calling for more research, plus Congress prohibiting federal interference in states' medical cannabis programs, more than a few centuries of **safe therapeutic use**, and a growing database of published research available (resulting from more and more states legalizing cannabinoids for medicinal and/or recreational use), most doctors still know little to nothing about cannabinoids and their potential health benefits. The encouraging news is that CBD with less than .03% THC is now available, as previously mentioned, and more people are now experimenting with and experiencing its benefits - including older individuals who suffer from the ailments already mentioned in this chapter.

To reiterate the importance of understanding the ECS and potential benefits that cannabinoids may offer us, I'll conclude this chapter with a brief excerpt from an article written by Peter Grinspoon, MD, a primary care physician, educator, and cannabis specialist at Massachusetts General Hospital and an instructor at Harvard Medical School;

Study of the ECS was initially focused on attempts to understand (and demonize) an illegal drug, but new research has since flourished into a far more broad-based exploration into what is an astoundingly intricate and far-reaching system by which our bodies learn, feel, motivate, and keep themselves in balance. We are truly at the dawn of an age of discovery of the ECS and the development of new medicines that may help alleviate some of the cruelest diseases that people (and animals) suffer from. I am incredibly excited to see what discoveries await us as we continue to untangle the mysteries of the ECS.

As Thomas Edison reminded us over a century ago, *"the simple truth is you cannot improve on nature."*

Part 3
Implementing An Effective
Functional Fitness Plan

CHAPTER 17

Essential Components

"Take care of your body.
It's the only place you have to live."

Jim Rohm

MAYBE YOU'RE A frequent flyer at the local gym, exercising on your own or engaging in group fitness classes on a regular basis. Or you prefer subscriptions to apps like Peloton for motivation and instruction. There is certainly no shortage of free instruction and advice available on the internet. You may even have your own gym at home that you prefer. And, of course, there are those of us who choose to walk or run or ride our bikes regularly as our preferred exercise. Whatever it may be, you have - I hope - seen by now that regular and consistent physical activity that includes muscular strength exercises is an absolute necessity if you wish to remain active through your lifespan and die young as old as you can. The previous chapters were meant to convince you *"why"* you should include regular physical activity into your daily routines. This chapter's purpose is to show you *"what"* should be included in your approach.

An exercise regimen focused upon functional fitness - defined here as any exercise performed to improve our ability to successfully move (meaning *"injury free"*) through our normal life activities - should include some basic components that will be addressed in this chapter. The goal is to maximize your return on the investment of time and energy that you choose to make each time you embrace your preferred activities, and to ultimately increase the enjoyment you derive from them. What's presented in this chapter are essential components of a functional fitness program. You may already be doing much or all of this. If so, good for you. If not, hopefully these basic principles - as daunting and complicated as they may initially appear to be - make sense to you. They've helped me. I'd like them to help you as well and believe that they will when done correctly.

To reiterate, functional fitness incorporates activities that prepare you for what you do in your everyday life and, ideally, to enhance your enjoyment of them while remain injury-free. For instance, a functional exercise could be a lunge with a rotational twist. In doing so, this helps when you reach into the upper cabinet for a glass or when you visit the grocery store and find yourself stretching up across your body for a large container of laundry detergent. This is an example of rotational movement and is one of three planes of motion we typically move through in the course of a day...if we're active human beings. If you play golf or tennis or pickle ball, those three sports clearly involve rotational movement. The latter two also require lateral movement. Think about it. Are you performing these kinds of movement patterns in your exercise regimen? Most people I observe working out at the gym often aren't. If your daily exercise consists solely of walking, then you're likely not. I'm emphasizing functional movement patterns that mimic movements made in an everyday **active** life. And planes of motion should be an integral part of your weekly routine.

So let's first start with the ways in which we move through space around us. Most of us exercise in what is known in the fitness world as the **sagittal plane**. We move in this plane when we're exercising essentially in a straight line - forward or backward, up or down - and this is typically observed on cardio machines like the elliptical trainer, stationary bike, or even treadmill. Lifting weights are generally performed in the sagittal plane as well, unless you are intentionally introducing rotation by doing alternate repetitions that rotate your midsection through the movement. This latter example brings us to the second plane of motion - the **transverse plane**. We operate in this plane when we rotate our torsos from one side to another, like when we reach up to the opposite side of our bodies to retrieve that container of detergent or swing through the tennis or golf or pickle ball. The third plane of motion is called the **frontal plane** and this is simply a fancy name that refers to lateral side-to-side movement, like when we're shuffling from "east to west" and vice versa in a game of tennis or pickle ball, as already noted. Of the three planes mentioned, it's the transverse plane that often triggers injuries because we're twisting in such a way that our bodies aren't prepared to do; thus, the lower back or shoulder injury.

By the way, if you're a walker, you can easily incorporate all three planes of motion in your route by sliding laterally from, say, one light pole to the next, and performing twisting motions to the next light pole. I encourage people I work with to walk backwards as well (make sure you look ahead before doing this). I've been told (anecdotally) that 100 steps backwards is equal to 1000 steps moving forward.

So what specific kinds of movement patterns should be included in your weekly regimen? You need to incorporate the *"magic seven"* movements - **pushing, pulling, squatting, lunging, hinging, balancing** and - of course - **rotation**. Each of these movement patterns should be included in your routine - not necessarily on the same day, but certainly at least two times weekly - if you're to prepare yourself for everyday living and playing your sport(s) while remaining injury-free. I'll provide examples of each in the next chapter.

Another critically important aspect of training is a concept called **stabilization.** What's this mean? It means that we have stabilizing muscles around joints at various points in our bodies and these need to be strong in order for us to move about without causing something to pull out of alignment and incite injury. As mentioned at the start of this chapter, this is a straightforward explanation in that a more detailed one would be a book by itself. Just know that most muscles can serve as both stabilizers and **prime movers**, depending upon what movement you are executing.

For example, standing on one leg while working the other leg through band movements has the standing leg serving as the stabilizer while the other leg serves as the prime mover. Switch legs and the roles reverse. Strengthening your abdominal complex is a prime example of stabilization. As I shared with you near the beginning of this book, this is how I addressed my back issues seven years ago and continue to work those stabilizing muscles each day. The saying *"You can't shoot a cannon from a row boat"* provides a metaphor for the importance of core stabilization. Strengthening your abdominal complex should be included in your **daily** regimen. I'll provide examples in the next chapter.

Just know this - using the exercise machines that have you sitting (not functional) while pushing or pulling against the machine through the **exact** plane of motion - never varying because the machine sets the angle for you (again, not functional) - will not activate the little stabilizing muscles around joints that guide the movement in real life because there is no need to control the weight and keep it in balance. The machines do this for you. Free weights - kettle bells, dumbbells, the functional trainer, TRX bands, resistance bands - provide real-life movement patterns that prepare you for **active** daily living, especially when performed on your feet. Body-weight exercises like pushups and squats do the same. Even better, performing movements on unstable surfaces will activate stabilizing muscles while providing an excellent challenge for your balance. Foam pads or a BOSU are examples of unstable surfaces. I will provide an example of an exercise you can perform on each of those unstable surfaces in the next chapter.

Please note - exercise machines are clearly safe places to begin strength work because they don't require you to use proper lifting techniques...the machines do this for you. So, if you don't know how to use free weights, then it's wise to begin there. Having said this, I'd recommend hiring a personal fitness coach. I know, I'm biased. But it really can be a wise investment and not an expense if you find a coach who teaches you proper techniques, even in just a few sessions. A personal fitness coach may also be able to identify compensation patterns you've developed over the course of time - like leaning one way while squatting or even walking, or one foot pointing outward to compensate for a lower back issue. It's worth it for your own health and well-being. It really is.

An aside - I worked in a big box gym a few years ago that had what I called a playpen specifically dedicated to the senior citizens who were enrolled in the Silver Sneakers Program. Of course, because I was a personal trainer who was nearest in age to these participants, I was assigned the role of "playground director" for this area. I doubt you'll be surprised at this point in the book that it used to piss me off that the senior citizens were funneled into this area. The challenge for most, by far, was actually slipping into the seat of each machine and then extricating themselves from it. Although it was certainly better than doing nothing, none of this was functional, as I hope you can see by what's been presented in this chapter so far.

Let us next address **joint health**, an issue that affects most of us at some point or another in our lives. All joints possess a **stability** component. All joints also possess a **mobility** component, with mobility defined as the ability to move a joint through its **full range of motion** (keep this in mind when performing strength exercises). Mobility, by the way, should not be confused with flexibility. They're similar, for sure, but the latter is defined as moving a joint *passively* through its range of motion while the former involves *active* movement. You should know that some joints lean towards stability while others prefer mobility.

Mother nature designed the **human kinetic chain** in such a way that joints provide stability or mobility in an alternating fashion. Beginning at the feet, joints located in that region of the body primarily provide stability (keeping you stable while standing). Moving up the kinetic chain, our ankles provide mobility, our knees stability, our hips mobility, our lumbar spine (lower back) stability, our thoracic spine (upper back) mobility, our scapula stability, and our shoulders mobility. It's really important for you to know the primary function of each joint area. Knowledge of these should drive your exercise routine. Here's why.

Your fitness routine should emphasize movement patterns that bring your mobilizing joints through their full range of motion - your ankles, hips, thoracic spine, and shoulders. The shoulder, for example, is the most mobile joint in our bodies. You can move your shoulders in multiple directions (when healthy) and in ways that other joints in your body can't move. Because your shoulders are so mobile, however, they are also most susceptible to injury. This is why it's vitally important to move them through their full range of motion and to strengthen the stabilizing muscles around the shoulder joints in order for them to remain on track (poor posture, by the way, can lead to joint dysfunction in the shoulder region). When muscle imbalances develop around the shoulder joint (or any joint, for that matter), the joint is pulled out of alignment and uneven wear and tear can occur.

Recall several chapters back when I mentioned our joints can remain with us for a lifetime if we take proper care of them. When we don't, then the uneven wear and tear eventually leads to surgery and/or a replacement (inborn anatomical imbalances can also contribute to this - I have a bowed leg greater on one side than the other that creates a leg length difference and deal with it accordingly by placing a small heal lift on the shortened side. *"Old"* injuries that we have compensated for over the years can lead to muscle imbalances as well). How do you activate the small stabilizing muscles around the shoulder joint? Free weights, as already mentioned in this chapter, will do this. Shoulder machines won't, primarily because the machines provide the stabilization for you. It's another reason to learn how to perform these exercises correctly simply because it will better prepare you for everyday living while avoiding nagging injuries.

Here's another example of how stabilizing joints work in concert with mobility joints. If I were to ask you the one area of our bodies that presents the most discomfort and pain, my guess is that you would say it's our lower back. You're absolutely correct if you did say this. Back pain is the most searched body part on Google and by far. How does back pain develop? Our lumbar spine (lower back) is designed to hold up the weight of our bodies. It serves, as you just read, as a stabilizing joint…when we stand, bend over, or twist. With strong postural muscles (core strength of the abdominal and glute complexes) and flexible joints above and below the lumbar spine as well as execution of functional movement mechanics, our lower backs will work properly and remain pain free. It's when we lack strength in our stabilizers along with reduced flexibility in the joints above and below our lumbar spine that back pain arrives. Our lumbar spines, when lacking stabilizing strength along with the inflexibility of the joints above and below it, then become mobilizing joints - a role they're not designed to serve. And so it eventually complains to us...in the form of lower back pain.

Another area of our bodies that invites trouble when unattended to is our knees. In the same way that our lumbar spine is a stabilizing joint, so too are our knees. When the muscles attached to the knees are weak and/or imbalanced and the mobilizing joints above and below the knees (our ankles and hips) are weak as well, the knees don't track properly and, thus, wear unevenly (excess weight is a major contributing factor as well). I don't have to tell you what is often the solution, but I will, anyway - typically, it's a ligament or meniscus repair or a knee replacement. I mentioned at the beginning of this book that I have a meniscus tear and my training regimen includes strength development for every muscle that attaches to that knee - the quadricep muscles, hamstring muscles, calf muscles, and tibial muscles. In addition, I make sure that my hips and ankles remain strong. So far, so good for me.

This is, admittedly, a cursory overview of joint health and the role each plays - mobilizing or stabilizing - in our everyday activity. Just keep these principles in mind when doing your exercise routine and make an effort to care for them accordingly.

Let's return to the *"magic seven"* movements now that I mentioned a few pages back. The first two - pushing and pulling - represent a push-pull paradigm that you should also incorporate into your fitness routine. Without getting too technical here, know that muscles work in groups. They don't work in isolation. When you bench press or perform a push-up, for example, your chest muscles are the prime movers (agonists) while your triceps assist as synergistic muscles and your latissimus dorsi (lats) as well as posterior deltoids serve as brakes (antagonists). Meanwhile, you should be engaging your core musculature for stabilization sake. So this is clearly a group effort. Conversely, when you pull, as in performing lat pulldowns or conventional pull-ups, everything is reversed. In order to execute both movement patterns - pushing and pulling - you are using a muscle **group.** Other examples are bicep curls in conjunction with tricep pushes and quadricep extensions combined with hamstring curls. In each example, muscles are working together. So when, for example, your quadriceps muscles are too strong for your hamstrings, then you are susceptible to hamstring pulls. Muscles need to be evenly developed around joints, as already noted, and this is also the case with muscles working together. So, each time you push a weight, the next exercise should be pulling weight in the opposite direction.

Another factor to consider with strength training involves **repetitions and sets**. Start slowly and warm up sufficiently to get blood flow to the areas you're working. A basic formula for developing both muscle strength and endurance is to aim for three sets of 8-12 repetitions per exercise, once warmed up, with the weight you're pushing and pulling equal to about 65-70 percent of what you could otherwise do one time. The chosen weight should challenge you enough such that the last few reps require real effort. If you're not pushing or pulling sufficient weight to make you *uncomfortable* in those last few repetitions, then you won't make any strength gains. Remember the *"sweet spot"*? It applies here as well. After a few weeks, if not sooner, you will notice that it becomes easier to execute these exercises simply because protein synthesis has occurred; thus, your muscles have become stronger.

So what should you do? Add weight by a factor of ten percent. Otherwise, you'll *"maintain"* what you've developed but never progress (I really don't like this word when I hear individuals say they're just trying to *"maintain"* strength. Why?). I liken this to putting money in your checking account and maintaining a balance, all the meanwhile actually losing money due to a rise in inflation. If you play a sport and are in your season, then maintenance makes perfect sense.

With a **push-pull routine**, there is no need to wait for recovery on a specific exercise. Just move to the next exercise and return to the previous one after a minute or two. **Circuit training** can work as well with this. It's both efficient and effective, keeping your heart rate elevated, and getting a higher return on your investment of time and energy.

As for **recovery** in between days, allow yourself at least forty-eight hours per muscle group and preferably seventy-two hours if you really pushed yourself out of your comfort zone. Why? You get stronger in between workouts and not during them due to the protein synthesis occurring while your body repairs the micro-tears you've created and it lays down even more muscle fiber in the process. And speaking of protein, you should increase your protein intake to take into account the muscle development you hope to experience. Protein is needed for muscles to develop, while complex carbohydrates provide the energy to perform the exercises. As for soreness, you may experience some and this is referred to as DOMS - delayed onset muscle soreness. It's alright if you experience some soreness. Active rest, meaning gentle to moderate movement of those muscles, should help to reduce the soreness. On the other hand, soreness that is debilitating - like it prevents you from doing what you normally do - is not alright. Back off and seek treatment, if necessary, before resuming again.

Still another consideration is the **tempo** of your repetitions. When you initiate a push or a pull, you are generating force known as a **concentric lift**. Conversely, when you've reached full range of motion on that push or pull, your return to the starting point is known as an **eccentric lift**. In the latter, you are absorbing force. It's this latter lift - the eccentric one - that often gets short shrift. It shouldn't because this is actually where you can gain more strength. In other words, the lift isn't over when you extend yourself. The return is equally important. If you're clanging the weight on its return, then you're not in control of the movement and you've lost the benefits of eccentric lifting. You can *"power up or down"* on a lift. Just make sure you control the weight upon its return to the starting point.

Here's an example of eccentric repetitions generating strength gains. I will sometimes encounter an individual who will tell me that s/he can't do a *"real"* pushup; only a *"girly"* one. You know, doing them with knees in contact with the ground. I don't want them doing those simply because they're training their nervous systems to do that kind of pushup and not a *"real"* one. So I have the individual get into a plank position on all fours and slowly descend to the ground, doing the second half of a *"real"* pushup. Once there, s/he can then drop to the knees and repeat the movement pattern by getting up in plank position and lowering by a count of five again. This is a perfect way to develop strength. In two or three weeks time, with repeated practice every other day (remember - you get stronger in between workouts), a *"real"* pushup becomes doable...even more than one. It's true. I've seen it done. Several times.

Yet one more consideration is something called **HIIT**, an acronym for **high-intensity-interval training**. Recall I mentioned at the beginning of this book that we need to have moments that - literally - take our breath away. HIIT is an excellent way to rev up our metabolism and put ourselves in the **anaerobic threshold** (when we're breathing heavily). Typically, the intervals can come in the form of a 10 - 30 second intensified movement. This could be on any of the cardio machines, or when you're walking or jogging. Not only does it elevate your heart rate for cardiovascular health while juicing your metabolic rate, it requires activation of **fast-twitch muscles**...the muscles that produce more force and power, and which happen to be the fibers we lose as we age. If you're doing 30 minutes on a cardio machine, warm up for five minutes and then introduce short intervals in between the aerobic pace you may otherwise be maintaining. Aim to do this twice weekly, **after clearing this with your doctor.**

I encourage you to consider **cross-training**, particularly if you're one of these individuals who prefers to do one activity... like walking, running, or cycling. Not only will cross-training help you to avoid overuse injuries, it will stimulate your nervous system to recognize different movement patterns for everyday living. Remember - accidents occur when our nervous system doesn't recognize in time what muscles it needs to recruit to avoid whatever causes the accident. **Variability** - introducing different kinds of movement - help both with physical and cognitive health. Moreover, muscular strength development, particularly upper body strength, should be included for those of you who solely walk, run, or cycle.

Lastly, **pay attention to what you're doing.** Otherwise, what you're doing won't pay you back sufficiently. It's important to actually feel what you're experiencing, to monitor what you're sensing in order to gain more control over your body. We've already addressed how prescriptions and the like have a way of numbing us. We don't need to contribute to this numbness by being inattentive to what we're doing. What's this mean? Instead of reading a book or watching television to distract you from the boredom of riding the recumbent bike, pay attention to how your body is responding to the movement. And pay attention to the exercise. I absolutely understand - it can be exceedingly boring at first. But know that not only are you training your body, you're training your brain as well. Train it to perform the exercise correctly, experience what you're feeling, and you'll find that you can extend time on the exercise for a longer duration. It's how adaptation to exercise - or anything, for that matter - works.

In the end, implementing a functional fitness regimen that incorporates the principles addressed in this chapter and listed below will all lead to helping you enjoy what you really want to experience in life - living an active lifestyle, playing your favorite sports without injury, and doing this for a lifetime.

- perform each of the **seven magic movement patterns** two or three times weekly (not all on the same day) - push, pull, squat, lunge, hinge, balance and rotate. Be sure to perform each movement in an **athletic position**, meaning slightly flexed knees and an engaged core complex.

- execute movements through the **three planes of motion** especially focusing upon lateral and rotational movements.

- keep aware of joint functions - whether the joint is primarily a **mobilizer or stabilizer** - when you are doing your exercise routine.

- be conscious of **sets** (two or three sets of each exercise) and **repetition counts** (eight to twelve reps, with the last few especially challenging you without compromising form).

- be aware of **tempo**, meaning that the second half or return of the movement to its starting point is as equally important as the initial push or pull is.

- incorporate **HIIT** a couple of times weekly, **after clearing this with your doctor.**

In the next chapter, I'll provide examples of these basic movement patterns you should incorporate into your weekly regimen that will help increase your functional fitness.

CHAPTER 18

A Menu of Movement Options

"There is more wisdom in your body than in your deepest philosophy."

Nietzsche

IN THIS CHAPTER, I'll present examples of movement patterns that link directly to the principles addressed in the previous chapter. Several different *"tools"* could be used to perform these movements - barbells, dumbbells, kettle bells, medicine balls, TRX bands, a functional trainer, stability/physio ball, resistance bands, ankle/hip bands, and even your own body weight in many cases. For the sake of simplicity, I've chosen to use resistance bands, ankle/hip bands, and my own body weight to demonstrate these exercises. I'll suggest some inexpensive tools you may wish to consider purchasing if you don't care to pay for access to a gym at the conclusion of the chapter.

Please note - Consult with your doctor before performing these exercises and know that you are proceeding at your own risk.

The first exercise I'll introduce is a **standard plank**, one that has you up on all fours (on elbows and feet) and holding steady - parallel to the floor - for, ideally, at least sixty seconds. This is considered an isometric hold. If you find yourself sagging (butt begins sinking to the floor) or lifting your butt up higher than the parallel hold should be, then stop doing the exercise and record how long you did it successfully. I often use the word *"yet"* in situations like these - you simply can't do a sixty-second plank…yet. By adding that three-letter word to any of these exercises strongly suggests that you will be able to do them eventually…just not yet. If you can already perform a sixty-second hold, then look to increase the time incrementally.

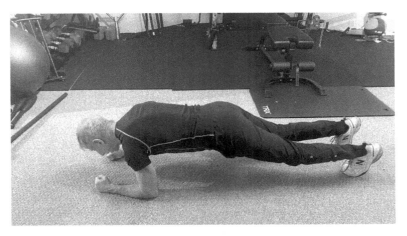

Standard Plank

Planks, and there are many variations, strengthen your **core muscles** - abdominal and lower back - that are designed to provide stability when moving other parts of your body. Recall shooting the cannon from the rowboat. You will increase your strength when you can better stabilize yourself during push and pull movements. Aim for a minimum of three planks each time you perform them, and not in succession. Rotate them through other exercises you are performing on that day. I've chosen this exercise first, by the way, because strong stabilization should precede any strength development regimen.

This next exercise is also an isometric hold, but in this case it activates your **oblique muscles**. These are especially important when rotating in the transverse plane - reaching up across your body to grab something or playing pickle ball, tennis, and golf. With this exercise, called a **side plank**, you turn to one side and lift your hips off the floor with a hand held high (again, there are variations of this exercise). Aim for thirty-second holds initially and look to increase the time as you become stronger at this. If you're not able to hold the side for thirty seconds *yet,* then hold it for as long as you can and then drop your hips to the floor and repeat until you reach a total of thirty seconds. Repeat on the opposite side. You should aim to perform this exercise at least three times weekly as well.

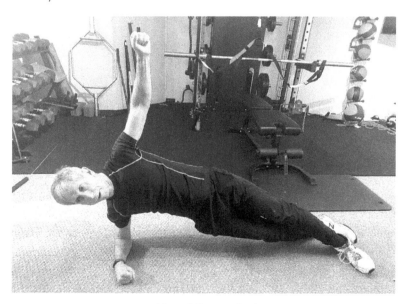

Side Oblique Plank

The third exercise selected is a **reverse plank** that activates your **posterior chain** otherwise known as your backside. Fully extend yourself on the floor with knees flexed and drive your heels into the floor or an elevated object. Just like the standard plank introduced as the first exercise in this chapter, you should aim to hold steady for sixty seconds. Pull out of it if you feel any unusual strain and repeat it until you reach the target time. Three times per workout is what you should eventually aim for.

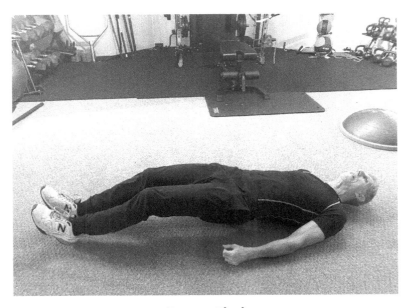

Reverse Plank

Next - anchor the resistance band to a safe and stable object. I've chosen to use a resistance band because you are far less likely to hurt yourself than you might with a dumbbell or kettle bell, especially if technique is an issue. We'll move into concentric and eccentric repetitions with these bands, beginning first with a **chest press**. This is considered a **push exercise**. Grab the handles at shoulder height and width, and push forward through the full range of motion. This means extending your arms until they're straight. Remember that tempo is important and make sure to control the movement to its return position. **Three sets of 8-12 reps should be your goal on this exercise and those that follow here.**

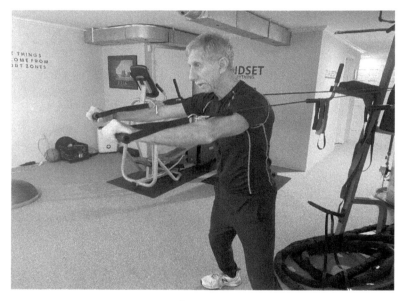

Chest Press

Remember the push-pull paradigm? Well, the next exercise should be a **pull movement**. So, in this case, you'll be doing three sets of **rows**. Turn yourself around to face the anchor point where the band is attached and pull the bands toward you until your hands reach your sides. Again, make sure to control the movement on its return to the starting position.

Your arms should be fully extended at the start of this exercise to make sure you're moving through a full range of motion.

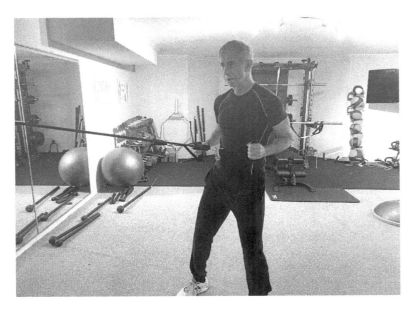

Row

Following the rows, you'll then focus upon your **triceps** by **push**ing them past your hips. Be certain to keep your palms facing down and arms relatively straight. Return each time to the starting position for full range of motion.

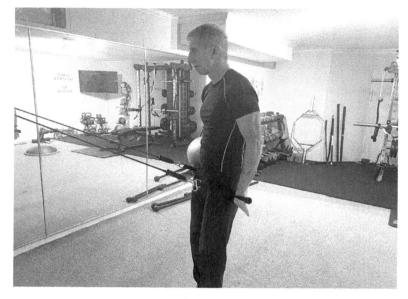

Tricep Push

You may already be able to figure out what's next in this sequence - it's a **bicep** curl. In this exercise, your palms should be facing up and you should hinge at your elbows while **pull**ing your hands to your face. Avoid pulling as if it's a row exercise. Stand far enough away from the anchor point to invite full range of motion and move just your arms, **hinging** at the elbows to activate your biceps.

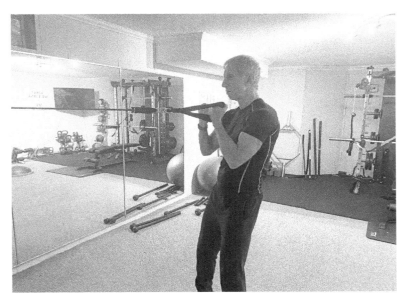

Bicep Curl

Next up is a **shoulder** press. Grab the handles of the band and place the band under your feet - the wider your feet are, the greater will be the resistance. Begin with your hands at shoulder height, p**ush** straight up to full extension and then return to the starting position under control.

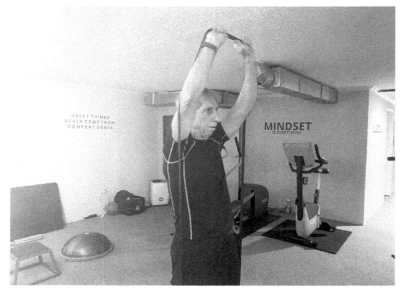

Shoulder Press

Follow the shoulder press with what's called an **upright row** where you will place your feet over the handles and **pull** the band up to your chin, activating your trapezoid muscles. You should notice the movement is directly opposite from what you executed with the shoulder press.

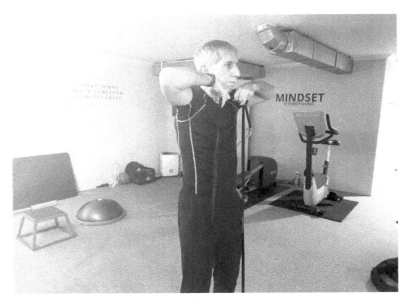

Upright Row

The next exercise will move you through the **frontal/lateral plane** of motion. Grab both handles and bring your hands together with arms extending forward at shoulder height. Take three steps out laterally from the anchor point and hold that position for thirty seconds. The larger the steps, the greater the challenge. Be certain to make each step equal in distance. When you begin your return in the opposite direction with three steps, make certain that the **leg closer to the anchor point** is the one you use to initiate that first return step. Returning to the starting point will require you to control the movement while keeping your balance. This is an excellent example of an **eccentric repetition** because you'll need to absorb the force of the pull while remaining under control. Repeat this movement on the other side.

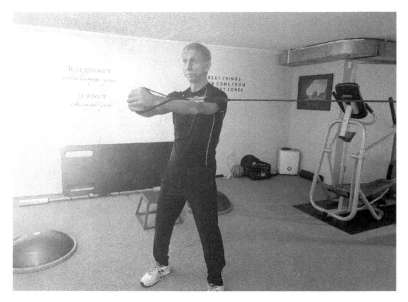

Lateral Three-Step Hold

Staying with your bands, this next movement will take you through the **transverse/rotational plane** of motion. This time you'll attach one handle to an anchor point (i.e., door knob) or you can simply tie the other handle to a stable object. Move yourself far enough away from the anchor point so that the arm connected to the handle is straight. Sweep your hand across your body while rotating through your midsection and then control the movement upon its return to the starting point. This exercise activates your **oblique muscles, chest muscles, and shoulder muscles** as well. The return will then bring in your rear deltoids (back of shoulder) in an eccentric rep. Repeat this with the other arm.

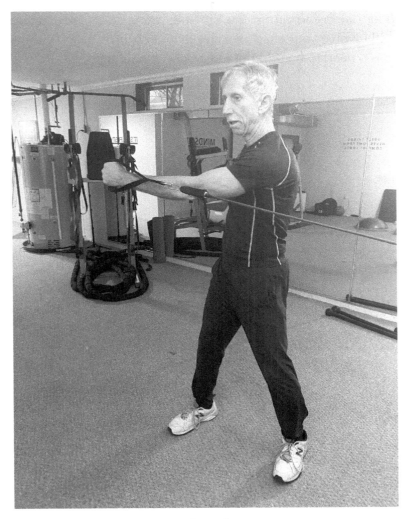

Chest Fly

Remaining in this position, now reach across your body to grab the handle with the hand farther away from the anchor point. This time you will repeat the sweeping motion, but you'll be activating your **rear deltoids and obliques** in

211

opposite fashion from the previous exercise and the return will involve your **chest muscles** in an **eccentric rep**, meaning you'll need to control the force upon the return.

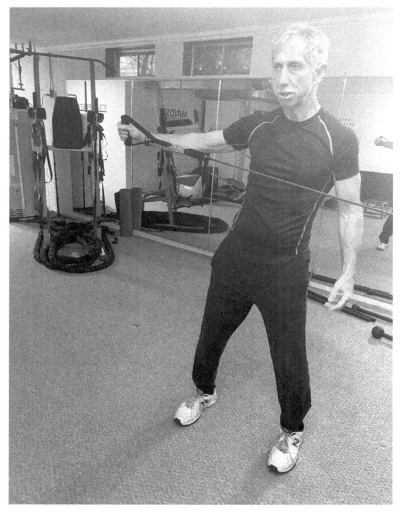

Reverse Fly

Each of these exercises focuses upon **upper body strength**. Aim to do these at **least two times weekly** and preferably three times. If done in succession, which they are sequenced for you to do, it should take about **thirty minutes to complete**. If this is cutting into your time walking, running, cycling or whatever, I believe it's time well spent. These exercises should also contribute to improved performance in your chosen activities.

We'll now move to your **lower body** and begin with a **body-weight squat**. Position your feet about shoulder width apart and place your hands near your chest. Descend to approximately a *ninety-degree angle* and then push through your heels to lift yourself back up to the starting position. By pushing through your heels, you'll activate your glute (butt) muscles, so you'll be using both your glutes and quadriceps in this exercise.

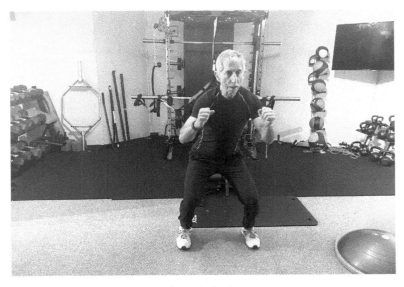

Body Weight Squat

I'm using an **ankle band** for this next exercise. Place the band around both upper ankles. If balance is a concern, do this alongside a wall or flat railing. The movement will be **lateral**, moving ten steps sideways and then retracing your steps to the starting point. The return should be ten steps as well. You should feel a burn in your glutes and hip flexors.

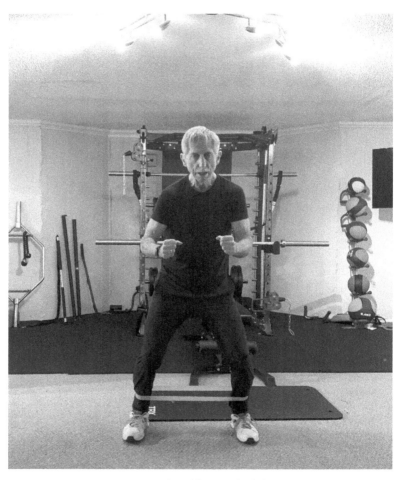

Lateral Ankle Band Slide

Moving on, the next exercise demonstrated is a reverse **lunge**. Begin in a standing position and then move one leg behind you while you flex your front leg in a lunge position. Alternate each leg for 8-12 repetitions.

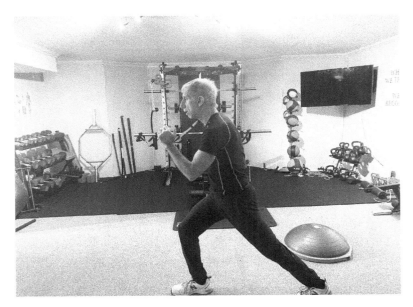

Reverse Lunge

This exercise will have you **hinging** at your hips. I'm using a kettlebell to demonstrate the exercise, but it could be any weighted object, even a basketball or soccer ball. Begin with the weighted object held in both hands with arms fully extended. Then initiate the exercise by swinging the ball through your legs, hinging at your hips, then pulling it back through and raising to about shoulder height. Repeat this for 8-12 repetitions.

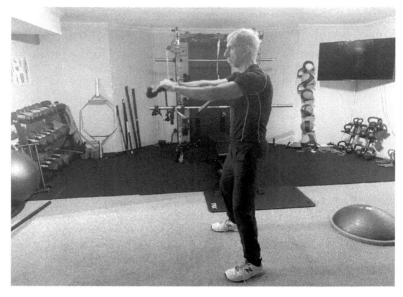

Hip Hinge

Next up is a single-leg **balance** exercise. You may want to position yourself next to a wall or some object you can touch if need be (but only if you must). Raise one leg and balance on the other. Aim for at least a **thirty-second** duration. Repeat on the opposite side. Increase your time standing without touching as you become more comfortable with this exercise.

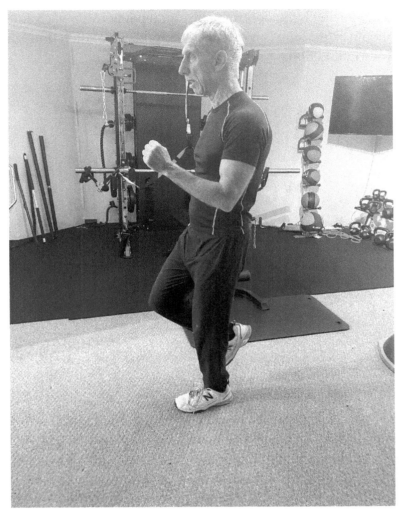

Single Leg Balance

I'll return to the second pull exercise you performed - a row. Now you'll perform this exercise **alternately**, reaching across and **rotating** your body. Alternate reps for each side, moving your right arm across on a 45-degree angle and then repeating with the opposite arm. Six repetitions on each side should be the aim. This exercise incorporates **rotation through your midsection**.

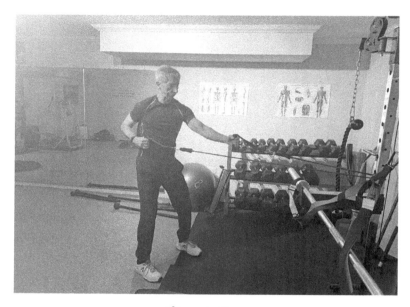

Alternate Rows

I'm combining the **alternate repetition**s on the **pull** with a rows while on an **unstable surfac**e - in this case it's a BOSU, but you may want to begin this on a foam pad when you're ready. By performing the exercise on an unstable surface, it will help with your balance while activating your core musculature to help you maintain your balance. When you're ready to increase the challenge, you can **perform any and all** of the push-pull sequenced exercises on an unstable surface.

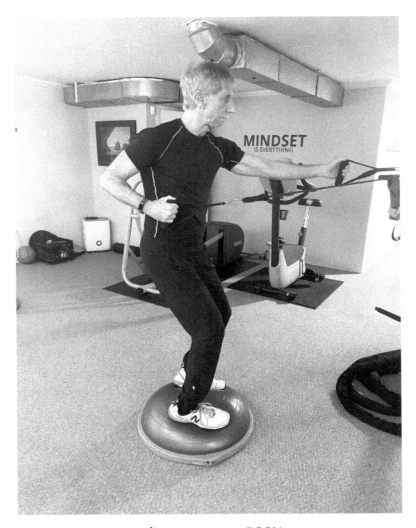

Alternate Row on BOSU

The final photo captures a few of the exercise tools you may wish to consider for use on a more regular basis.

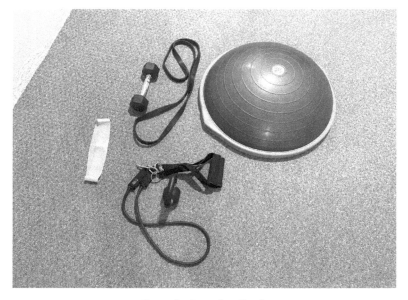

Sample Exercise Tools

Know that the exercises performed with the resistance band could easily be replicated on a functional trainer. With proper form and technique, they could be executed with dumbbells as well.

Please understand this is a program that includes the basic components of a functional fitness program, incorporating all of the principles touched upon in the previous chapter. As you become more adept at performing these exercises with a resistance band, you most definitely should consider using other tools to advance your fitness.

Remember - muscles matter. Work them regularly and they will serve you well.

PART 4
ROLE MODELS & REFLECTIONS

CHAPTER 19

Role Models

"We tend to become like those we admire."

Thomas Monson

I'VE ALWAYS HAD role models. As a young kid, they were Whitey Ford and Willie Mays. Lenny Wilkens and Bob Cousy. Jerry West and Mickey Mantle. My baseball cards? They were precious gold to me (they'd be, literally, precious gold today if I knew where they were). When I graduated to middle school, my role models got closer to me geographically - the local high school stars I wanted to emulate and, indeed, tried to whenever I stepped on the basketball court or baseball diamond. And, of course, there were my UConn heroes I admired so much as well. I stood in the batter's box just like they would, delivered pitches with the same windup, moved around the basketball court and shot the ball with the same form they used...or so I thought. There were countless times when, either out in my backyard or alone at the park basketball courts, I would deliver the final pitch against the chimney and strike out the last batter to win the World Series or make the last second shot to capture the NBA championship.

With my own imagination at play, I was the radio announcer describing the action that I - the player - was performing. Of course, I always won, even if I had to repeat the scenario a few times to get it *"right"*. I doubt I was any different than most kids, especially those who were enamored with sports like I was.

As I grew older, my idols changed. I wanted to be more like the veteran teachers who delivered lessons with enthusiasm and humor, who inspired and cared about what they did…who genuinely supported their students. I wanted to be like the coaches I had and whom I looked up to for fatherly advice. Most of all, I wanted to be like my parents when I became one myself. Imitation, it's been said, is the sincerest form of flattery. It was certainly the case with my heroes. All of them.

And so now as I've grown older and I'm moving through the eighth decade of my life, I find myself searching for role models who are out in front of me, meaning older than I am. People who continue to embrace life with a full vigor and passion, who squeeze the juice out of the lemons handed to them - the lemons delivered to us all with the passage of time - and who seek joy in everything that's around them. Like E. E. Cummings advised us, *"It takes courage to grow up and become who you really are."* I've found some role models to emulate, and I'll continue to find more along the way.

Some of these role models are individuals I've worked with in my role as a personal fitness coach. There were Doc and Bill, both in their late eighties and college roommates back in their day, who would enthusiastically walk together into the gym and encourage each other as one performed an exercise while the other waited his turn. Doc was a *"character"* - he checked himself out of an assisted-living facility because he refused to use the walker they required when he moved about the premises. This is the same guy who, when he first set foot on a BOSU, could balance himself for just three seconds before needing to grab hold of one of the two bicycle handles adjacent to the BOSU. Three months later, Doc was standing on that same BOSU for forty-three seconds before needing to touch that handle. And Bill, when we first measured his stride length (remember - I referred to stride length as a preliminary indicator of cognitive decline), needed eighty-eight steps to cover the designated distance we established. Three months later, he covered the same distance in sixty-eight steps.

Then there was Mary, an 81-year old woman visiting her daughter one summer and who came to the gym looking for some help with her fitness. Somehow, we found each other. When I asked her what she was hoping to achieve in her fitness sessions that summer, she told me she *"wanted to get up higher on the mountain."* Needing clarification, I asked her what she meant. She told me she was a skier and she wanted to begin her runs higher up the trail. So, we went back to the trusted BOSU, eventually flipping it once she became more comfortable with it, and put ski poles in her hands to simulate the movement of skiing down the mountain. She was a warrior.

Barry is still another role model I look to for hope and inspiration. A gritty 82-year-old gentleman with a hard-nosed mentality, he worked his way up through the ranks of corporate life, beginning as a gas attendant while in high school and eventually rising to become a top executive in the very company he first pumped gas for. He arrives at the gym each time with a can-do attitude and moves through each exercise routine with determination and commitment, doing it all in a manner I hope to be emulating in a decade or so when I reach that age.

I've found other role models online, a couple of whom I'll share with you before we close out this book. Willie Spruill is one example among many I've discovered. A typical kid growing up several decades ago when kids played outdoors most of the day, he played baseball through high school and then enlisted in the army because he couldn't afford to attend college. He loved the physical nature of the military until one particular assignment changed everything for him. *"While I was in the army, I cracked my spine and my pelvis jumping out of an aircraft,"* he said. *"It was tough. For a guy who likes to be out and involved you can't really do much of anything, and in my case, things only got worse instead of better.".*

In chronic pain, he visited several doctors trying to find a remedy. But the pain only seemed to get worse, to the point where he couldn't walk without a cane. *"What made things even worse is I was on all these prescription medications, all these narcotics, and I couldn't think clearly,"* said Spruill. *"I wasn't me anymore. I was confused, frustrated, suffering and couldn't see it ever getting better."*

Then it just so happened that he came across a brochure advertising the North Carolina Senior Games. *"It was like for just a second the old me shined through. So, I went over to the track and started walking, one painful step at a time."* And it was there on the track, immersed in an athletic environment and being around others who were working out, that something triggered in him the desire to move like he once did.

"The first thing I did was throw that cane down and I started walking," he said. *"Started doing it every day. Pushed a little, then pushed a little more. After a few weeks I got to where I tried for more. And to my surprise I can remember screaming out, "I can run again. I can run again."* Willie soon starting cutting back on his pain medications and found himself thinking more clearly, pushing through the agony until it eventually subsided. Soon, his confidence grew and he decided to enter into three events in the Senior Games. Guess what? He won them all.

Willie is not without pain these days. He still suffers from sciatica and migraine headaches, painful enough to keep him temporarily sidelined. Yet, when he's able, he gets back on the track right away. *"This is my sanctuary,"* said Spruill. *"This is where I find strength and peace. Being out here on the track surrounded by all these people over 50 with all this positive energy, I can't go wrong. I cannot go wrong. The Senior Games gave me my life back."* Spruill goes on to say, *"Sometimes it brings me tears when I think about it, what I have been through and what I have had to overcome. And it's still not over. There are still certain times of the year where if I twist wrong, I might end up bent over again. But I know I'm going to get up, get back out there and I'm going to strive every day to motivate every person I see."*

I never met Willie Spruill in person but would certainly love to some day…perhaps at a Senior Games down the road. He may not know it, but his story is inspiring for me. I hope it is for you as well.

One more *"senior citizen"* I'll highlight here, and there are many more I've found in the course of my searches that I wish I could include but space and time won't allow, is a 94-year-old grandmother. Colleen Milliman is her name. Back in 2017, one of her grandchildren challenged her to get on a track and see what she could do. So, she did. And, indicative of her intent, she brought a stopwatch with her. *"I did it just to amuse him,"* Milliman said. *"Turns out, I am fast."*

Shortly thereafter, she registered for the Hayward Classic, a local run, simply to participate and discover what she could do. Well, she found out she could set world records. She established a new benchmark of 13 minutes and twenty-six seconds. *"I had no idea I would set a record. It was something new to do and try,"* she said. *"It was the very first time I ran a mile at Hayward Field and it turned out to be a record."* She also became the oldest woman to ever officially race a mile. Colleen wasn't finished, though. She went on to also break the Women's over-90 age group in the 800 meter race in a time of five minutes and forty-four seconds, eclipsing the previous record by one minute and twelve seconds.

Milliman continued to be active and took pleasure in meeting other athletes. She told anyone who was willing to listen that growing old is mandatory, growing up is optional, but laughing at yourself is therapeutic. *"Most of the time people think they are too old at 60 or 70 and they stop doing things,"* Milliman said. *"Well, I guess I'm selfish and I don't like to feel old. I stay active and I laugh at myself a lot."*

Milliman was always active prior to her newfound track career, walked regularly around her neighborhood. It wasn't until after she set her first record that she motivated herself to staying even more active by eating healthy, joining a gym, and entering meets. Colleen still hopes that others will also seek motivation to pursue what's important to them. Although she doesn't see herself as a role model, still she said, "*I want everybody to try to be positive and not be negative. If you do that it's always better. Things don't always turn out the way you want them to but it would be worse if you didn't try to make it better.* " Remember that *National Poll on Healthy Aging* presented way back in Chapter Two? Our attitudes go a long way in determining how we feel and what we can do as we age.

She may not see herself as an inspiration to others, but that doesn't mean that I have to agree with her. She's most certainly an inspiration to me.

Like all of the preceding examples shared here, they provide hope for what's possible up ahead...if we stay on our feet and keep moving. It's the essential theme of this book... physical activity, more than anything else, will go a long way in helping you die young as old as you can.

CHAPTER **20**

Conclusion

***Just when the caterpillar thought the world was
over, it became a butterfly.***

A Proverb

THIS BOOK HAS been a passion project of mine, initially
born from the accident I referred to in the Foreword, but it's
one that has likely been percolating for several years, anyway.
It just had to take an obstacle - that accident - to finally get
me to move forward with it. To bring this to fruition and arrive here at what I've decided is its conclusion has had me
experience a range of emotions as I've reflected upon the past
seven decades of my life, reflections I don't typically make
because I prefer to set my sights on what's in front of me.
Rear-view mirrors don't work for me. But it's been necessary
for me to look there and, in so doing, this passion project has
evolved into a personal narrative more than any attempt at
constructing some semblance of an academic treatise. Thus,
the fond memories and the not-so-fond ones, the trials, the
tribulations, the lessons learned along the way in the course
of my seventy-two years of living, have had me writing from

my heart more than from my head. Passion has a way of doing this simply because passion does originate in the heart, if not the soul.

Having said that, it was never my intention to simply share my personal experiences. My intention has been to weave in legitimate research evidence to support the narrative I wished to convey. I hope I've done this for you.

I've never written a book before, unless you count a dissertation as a book. I don't. A dissertation, if you've ever written or read one, is formulaic - five chapters laid out in basically a template form and written in what I like to call *"journalese"* prose. I had no template here. I preferred it this way because, remember, I'm a contrarian by nature. It just made it more challenging to do. It also made it more rewarding for me in the end. Back to my home gym one more time, I have a saying posted on a wall that reads *"If it doesn't challenge you, it won't change you."* This wasn't my primary objective, but the challenge in writing this book has fundamentally changed me going forward in my life…and, I sincerely believe, for the better. I hope that it changes you for the better in some way as well.

I've made my best-faith effort to provide research support for the beliefs I've expressed here, and I've made a similar effort in documenting these resources so the reader knows from where they came. With that said, I may have missed a reference here or there along the way and I apologize for this if I have. Just please know this - I don't believe, in Kathryn Strong's word referred to back in Chapter 10, that I was *"confabulating"* at any point in the book. I made every effort to not avoid letting the facts get in the way of my narrative and, instead, let the facts support it. The references are made in the context of my writing. They're listed at the end of the book as well. To reiterate, I may have missed one or two or three and, if I have, I'm telling you now. Mea culpa.

Beginning anything from a fresh start is never easy. It just takes consistent effort on a daily basis until you begin to feel as though you've created a body of something you believe is alive and real. We addressed this back in Chapters 12 and 13 with habit formation. When the challenges became difficult, I turned to my *"why"* for writing this in order to help me push through or around or over the obstacles I faced along the way. And, indeed, there were obstacles along the way. But we learned that the obstacle **is** the way in Chapter 15. I believe these obstacles, in the end, helped me to write this book to its conclusion.

Now it's your turn. No matter where you are in your personal journey, it's never too late to start. You still have much to live for, so many moments to experience, so much joy to behold and - yes - so many challenges to face, particularly as you move through each passing decade. Believe me, I know. If you think it's over and not possible for you to grow any more in your later years, please hold on to this proverb for strength and perseverance - ***Just when the caterpillar thought the world was over, it became a butterfly.***

Thank you so much for listening.

Epilogue

SO - YES - I wrote this book, but many others were major contributors to this venture in their own ways. I'm sure you'll agree that nobody achieves anything solely by their own doing. I have several people to thank and I wish to do so here in this space, knowing full well that I may miss acknowledging someone that deserves recognition.

I have my older brother, Rich, to thank for allowing me to tag along with him as a pip squeak in the housing project with the older kids when it would have been so much easier for him to leave me behind. I shared my childhood experience playing with the older project kids in the first chapter. I couldn't have done this without him. He looked out for me and made sure I got into the games they played…and there were so many to play. Those were very formative years for me and I have him to thank for this.

I have my younger sister, Joanne, to thank as well for being my soul mate, especially through the third and fourth and fifth decades of my life. She was and continues to be both a sounding board and reassuring voice for me. We have always had a shared perspective about life, with nuanced differences that have allowed me to learn from her and help me grow forward. She remains so to this day.

I wish my college basketball coach and lifelong mentor, Dee Rowe, was alive today for me to share this book with him. When I completed my dissertation defense at UConn several years ago, it was his office on campus that I went to first in order to share the news. He was like a father to me, especially after my father passed away, and he still is a source of inspiration for me today even in his passing.

I've already shared with you in the chapter on Role Models that I hoped to be the kind of parent for my children that my mother, Rosalind, and my father, Walter, were to me. One an Italian and the other Irish, they were a perfect blend. Each, in their own unique ways, encouraged me to take chances, to find out what I could do, and to fail along the way without judgement. They were so supportive in all that I pursued, and they were there by my side - either literally or in spirit - every step of the way in my journey. I wish, too, they were alive today to share this with them. I think of them every day and will so for the rest of my life.

Now that I'm grateful for having the opportunity to be a parent, I've been blessed to share my life with three incredible children - Luke, Dan, and Anthony. As much as I have tried to be the parent for them that my parents were to me, each son has given back to me and taught me lessons about life that I'll need to someday put into words for them to understand.

Finally, I have my wife, Eileen, to thank...I'm not sure where to begin or where it would even end...for being the steadying force for me as I've often wobbled through this life as the contrarian that I am. For thirty-seven years, she has endured my sometimes rebellious spirit, always being the patient and caring soul that she truly is. I would not have completed this passion project if not for her guiding support along the way. For this, I am certain. Absolutely certain.

References

Chapter 2

Experiences of Everyday Ageism and the Health of Older US Adults: Julie Ober Allen, PhD, MPH; Erica Solway, PhD, MSW, MPH; Matthias Kirch, MS; et al., *JAMA Network Open*. 2022

National Data on Age Gradients in Well-Being Among US Adults *JAMA Network Open, August 2022*

https://www.ssa.gov/history/age65.html

Chapter 3

https://thischairrocks.com/

https://www.ted.com/talks/ashton_applewhite_let_s_end_ageism 2017

Why Do We Age?

A question almost as old as time
By Brooke Borel | Published Mar 30, 2016 in *Popular Science*

The Wear and Tear Theory of Aging By Mark Stibich, PhD medically reviewed by Jenny Sweigard, MD
Very Well Health Updated on September 04, 2022

Why Do We Age? Four Theories of Aging by J.P. March 22, 2021 *Longevity Advice*

Study Confirms that Some People Age More Slowly Amy Norton *UPI* March 19, 2021

Cracking the Aging Code Josh Mitteldorf Dorion Sagan 2017 Flatiron Books New York

What Is Epigenetics Theory? by Julia A. Fast, medically reviewed by Jerry Kennard, Ph.D. in *Very Well Health,* August 2019

Chapter 4

The World Health Organization (WHO) Approach to Healthy Aging by Ewa Rudnicka, Paulina Napierala, Agniescka Podfigurna, Blasej Meczakalski, Roman Smolarczyk, and Monika Grymowicz: Published online 2020 May 26. doi: j. maturis. 101016/j. maturitas. 2020.05.018

Baltimore Longitudinal Study On Aging https://www.blsa.nih.gov/

https://www.susanflory.com/nadia-tuma-weldon/

Episode 14: Colin Milner, Founder & CEO, International Council on Active Aging (ICAA) MFN/ 20 August 2020/Podcast/

Live Long Master Aging Podcast
Paul Irving, Episode 10: Promoting purposeful aging & fighting for older people

Longevity Increased by Positive Self-Perceptions of Aging: Becca R. Levy, Martin Slade, Suzanne R. Kunkel, Stanislav V. Karl in *Journal of Personality and Social Psychology* August 2002

Head First: The Biology of Hope and the Healing Power of the Human Spirit by Norman Cousins, January 1989 published by Dutton Books

Study Confirms that Some People Age More Slowly by Amy Norton *HealthDay News* reported in UPI March 19, 2021

Chapter 5

Americans give health care system failing mark: AP-NORC poll reported by Amanda Seitz, September 12, 2022 in https://www.yahoo.com/news/americans-health-care-system-failing-041951858.html

Mayo Clinic Back Surgery: When Is It a Good Idea? https://www.mayoclinic.org/diseases-conditions/back-pain/diagnosis-treatment/drc-20369911

5 Common Medications That Can Cause Weight Gain *AARP* https://www.aarp.org/health/drugs-supplements/info-2022/medication-weight-gain.html

National Health and Nutrition Examination Survey
National Center for Health Statistics; NCHS Fact Sheet, July 2020

https://www.msn.com/en-us/health/medical/use-of-ibuprofen-could-increase-risk-of-chronic-pain-study-shows/

Medication Overload and Older Americans
https://lowninstitute.org/projects/medication-overload-how-the-drive-to-prescribe-is-harming-older-americans/

Over-the-Counter Relief From Pains and Pleasures Alike: Acetaminophen Blunts Evaluation Sensitivity to Both Negative and Positive Stimuli by Jeffrey R. O. Durso, Andrew Luttrel, and Baldwin M. May in *Sage Journals Association for Psychological Science* Volume 26 Issue 6

US FDA: Why You Need to Take Your Medications as Prescribed or Instructed; Center for Disease Control COVID Tracker
https://covid.cdc.gov/covid-data-tracker/#datatracker-home

Tackling the Growing Problem of Overmedication: *Knowable Magazine* https://knowablemagazine.org/article/health-disease/2021/tackling-growing-problem-of-overmedication

Addressing the unique care needs of older adults: *Age Friendly Health Systems* https://www.aha.org/center/age-friendly-health-systems

U.S. Health in International Perspective: Shorter Lives, Poorer Health: National Library of Medicine: https://www.ncbi.nlm.nih.gov/books/NBK154489/

The NIH director on why Americans aren't getting healthier, despite medical advances Selena Simmons-Duffin Podcast *NPR* December 7, 2021

Too Many Prescription Drugs Can Be Dangerous, Especially for Older Adults: https://publichealth.hsc.wvu.edu/media/3331/polypharmacy_pire_2_web_no-samhsa-logo.pdf

Chapter 6

https://www.usda.gov/media/blog/2014/05/27/100-years-tracking-nutrients-available-us-food-supply

Suzette Pereira Ph.D. https://thedoctorweighsin.com/author/spereira/

Why Some Doctors Let Patients Skip Weight Checks: *Wall Street Journal* Sumathi Reddy March 7, 2022

Is It Time To Move On From BMI? The Atlantic, RE; Think Original Sponsored by Abbott Laboratories

What Is Body Composition? *Very Well Health* by Ashley Braun MPH, RD July 13, 2022 Medically Reviewed by Ashley Baumohl MPH, RD

Gait Speed and Survival in Older Adults Stephanie Studenski, MD, MPH; Subashan Perera, PhD; Kushang Patel, PhD; et al *JAMA Network* January 5, 2011

Poor handgrip strength in midlife linked to cognitive decline September 1, 2022 by Heidi Godman, Executive Editor, Harvard Health Letter

Grip strength can indicate your cause of death by Thea Myklebust August 2016 sciencenorway.no

Highlights of Research Results from the Kuakini Honolulu Heart Program and Kuakini Honolulu-Asia Aging Study; Longevity and Health Survival: https://www.kuakini.org/wps/portal/kuakini-research/research-home/in-the-news/highlights-of-kuakini-research-results June 23, 2022

Associations Between Handgrip Strength and Dementia Risk, Cognition, and Neuroimaging Outcomes in the UK Biobank Cohort Study by Kate A. Duchowny Ph.D., Sarah F. Ackley, Ph.D., Willa D. Brenowitz, Ph.D. et al

Association Between Push-up Exercise Capacity and Future Cardiovascular Events Among Active Adult Men *JAMA Open Network* February 2019 by Justin Yang, Costas A. Christophi, Andrea Farioli, Dorothee M. Bower, Steven Moffat, Terrel M. Zollinger, Stefanos N. Kales

The Power of One Push-Up by James Hamblin *The Atlantic* June 27, 2019

Chapter 7

Want to Know Your Biological Age? Buyer Beware.
No matter what age tests reveal, experts say the real key to longevity is exercise By Kerri Miller in *Next Avenue* August 29, 2022

Why is life expectancy in the US lower than in other rich countries? by Max Roser 10/29/20 in *Our World In Data*

How Old Are You Really? Meet Your 'Biological Age' by Betsy Morris May 24, 2022 in the *Wall Street Journal*

Slowing down aging: the telomerase track? *In Encyclopedia of the Environment;* https://www.encyclopedie-environnement. org/en/zoom/slowing-down-aging-the-telomerase-track/

Should you be tested for inflammation?March 29, 2022 By Robert H. Shmerling, MD, *Harvard Health Publishing*

Inflammaging: chronic inflammation in aging, cardiovascular disease, and frailty Luigi Ferrucci and Elisa Fabbri July 31, 2018 *Nature Reviews Cardiology*

Why all the buzz about inflammation — and just how bad is it? March 16, 2022 by Robert H. Shmerling, MD, *Harvard Health Publishing*

Effect of Comprehensive Lifestyle Changes on Telomerase Activity and Telemere Length in Men With Biopsy-Proven Low Risk Prostate Cancer: Five-Year Follow-up of a Descriptive Pilot Study Prof Dean Ornish, MD et al
The Lancelot Oncology September 17, 2013

Chapter 8

Exercise Controls Gene Expression Frank W. Booth and P. Darrell Neufer in *American Scientist* Volume 93

The Unseen Role Our Muscles Play In Getting Older *The Atlantic* Re: Think Original https://www.theatlantic.com /sponsored/ensure-2017/the-unseen-role-our-muscles-play-in-getting-older/1350/

Preserve Your Muscle Mass Feb 19, 2016 *Harvard Health Publishing*

Age and Muscle Loss Nov 11, 2021 *Harvard Health Publishing*

Older People Must Work Out More to Keep Muscles by Matt McMillen, Reviewed by Laura J. Martin Jul8, 2011 *WebMD*

Pilegaard, H., G. A. Ordway, B. Saltin and P. D. Neufer. 2000. Transcriptional regulation of gene expression in human skeletal muscle during recovery from exercise. *American Journal of Physiology: Endocrinology and Me- tabolism* 279

Gabrielle Lyon *Muscular Medicine* https://drgabriellelyon.com/

John Morley, MD https://medfaculty.slu.edu/details/2874/john-morley

Chapter 9

Kay Bowman Author *Move Your DNA* Propriometrics Press; 1st edition (October 15, 2014)

The Economics of Obesity By Tomas J. Philipson June 28, 2022 *Wall Street Journal*

Physical activity definition by the *National Library of Medicine*

Non-exercise activity thermogenesis James A. Levine *Mayo Clinic* Published - Aug 2003

Walking for Fitness Mayo Clinic April 22, 2021 *Mayo Clinic*

Do you really need to walk 10,000 steps a day? Here's what experts say by Kaitlin Reilly *Yahoo Life* May 31, 2022

Chapter 10

Piaget's Stages: 4 Stages of Cognitive Development and Theory; Any Child Psychology textbook you prefer

Being Wrong: Adventures in the Margin of Error by Kathryn Schulz 2011 HarperCollins Publishers

Chapter 11

Start with Why: How Great Leaders Inspire Everyone to Take Action Simon Sinik October 2009

Find Your Why: A Practical Guide for Discovering Purpose for You and Your Team by Simon Sinik 2017 Portfolios Publishing

Chapter 12

Good Habits, Bad Habits byWendy Wood, 2020 Picador Paper

Mastery: The Keys to Success and Long-Term Fulfillment by George Leonard 1992 Plume Publishing

The Fifth Discipline: The Art and Practice of The Learning Organization by Peter Senge 2006 Doubleday

Atomic Habits by James Clear 2018 Avery Publishing

How Long Does It Take for a New Behavior to Become Automatic? https://www.healthline.com/health/how-long-does-it-take-to-form-a-habit

Breaking Bad Habits August 13, 2021 *Psychology Info*

Man's Search for Meaning by Victor Frankl 2006 Beacon Press

Dopamine: The Pathway to Pleasure July 20, 2021 Stephanie Watson *Harvard Health Publishing*

Breaking Bad Habits: Why It's So Hard to Change Jan 2012 *NIH News In Health*

Chapter 13

The Science of Forming Healthy Habits by Theresa Sullivan Barger *Discover* Jan 3, 2022

Why Only 8% of People Achieve Their Goals, According to Research Max Phillips Sept 14 2020 Published in *Ascent Publication*

New Year's Resolutions Statistics August 2022 Discover Happy Habits https://discoverhappyhabits.com/new-years-resolution-statistics/

The Power of Habit: Why We Do What We Do in Life and Business by Charles Duhigg 2012 Random House

The Craving Mind by Judson Brewer 2018 Yale University Press

Tiny Habits: The Small Changes that Change Everything by B. J. Fogg 2021 Harvest Publishing

Chapter 14

The Sweet Spot: The Pleasures of Suffering and the Search for Meaning by Paul Bloom 2021 Ecco Publishing

Benign Masochism: The Theory That Explains Why You Enjoy Chillies, Depressing Music, and Rollercoasters in *Esquire* 2016

Switch: How to Change Things When Change Is Hard by Chip Heath and Dan Heath 2010 Crown Business Publishing

Chapter 15

The Obstacle Is the Way: The Timeless Art of Turning Trials into Triumph by Ryan Holliday 2014 Portfolio Publishing

Chapter 16

Medical Cannibas by Jon O. Ebbert, MD, MsC, Eugene L. Scharf MD, Ryan T. Hurt MD, Ph.D *Mayo Clinic Proceedings, Concise Review for Clinicians,* Volume 93, Issue 12, December 1, 2018

The Endocannabinoid System: Essential and Mysterious by Peter Grinspoon, *Harvard Health Publishing*, August 11, 2021

What Is the Endocannabinoid System? by Adrienne Dellwo, Medically Reviewed by Jenny Sweigard, MD *Very Well Health*, February 10, 2020

The Health Effects of Cannabis and Cannabinoids: The Current State of Evidence and Recommendations for Research (2017) *The National Academy of Sciences, Medicine Engineering: The National Academies Press*

Committee on the Health Effects of Marijuana: An Evidence Review and Research Agenda; Board on Population Health and Public Health Practice; Health and Medicine Division; National Academies of Sciences, Engineering, and Medicine, National Academies of Sciences, Engineering, and Medicine 2017. The Health Effects of Cannabis and Cannabinoids: The Current State of Evidence and Recommendations for Research. Washington, DC: *The National Academies Press*. https://doi.org/10.17226/24625.

Chapter 17

National Academy of Sports Medicine Essentials of Corrective Exercise Manual for Personal Fitness Trainers; Edited by Michael A. Clark, Scott C. Lucett, Brian G. Sutton; 2014 Jones & Bartlett Learning

Built From Broken: A Science-Based Guide to Healing Painful Joints, Preventing Injuries, and Rebuilding Your Body by Scott Hogan, CPT, COES 2021 Salt Wrap Publishing

Chapter 18

National Academy of Sports Medicine Essentials of Corrective Exercise Manual for Personal Fitness Trainers ; Edited by Michael A. Clark, Scott C. Lucett, Brian G. Sutton; 2014 Jones & Bartlett Learning

Chapter 19

Willie Spruill Finds Sanctuary on the Track : *Growing Bolder*
https://growingbolder.com/stories/willie-spruill-finds-sanctuary-on-the-track/

*S*peeding Up At 94, Eugene Civic Alliance, February 3, 2021

About the Author

DOUG MELODY IS a lifelong educator who has served in a variety of roles during a 46-year career in the profession, teaching at every level from kindergarten to graduate school and each grade level in between. With a Ph.D. in Educational Psychology, a dissertation completed in the area of sport performance, several certifications in the fitness field, a lifetime of working out in - literally - hundreds of gyms, and collaborating with scores of individuals in their quest to become more fully functioning human beings, Doug is now sharing his knowledge and experience with the hope that readers can begin to shape a new narrative on how to grow older in healthier ways. We can do better and this book is an attempt to explain both why and how we can do this.

CPSIA information can be obtained
at www.ICGtesting.com
Printed in the USA
BVHW061910131222
654115BV00004B/17